ADVANCE PRAISE FOR
DELUSIONS, MEANING AND TRANSFORMATION

"*Delusions, Meaning, and Transformation* is a ground breaking book that is accessible, hopeful, and immensely useful. I have waited a long time for a book that provides such in depth yet accessible knowledge about the experience of psychosis as well as powerful strategies that can be utilized in a helping role."

— Sharon Young, Ph.D. CooperRiis Institute Director, CooperRiis Healing Community

"Milt Greek has produced an inspiring and inspired piece of work that that allows the reader the privilege to 'hear' the voices and 'read' the minds of individuals who often become relegated to the margins of society due to their mental afflictions. It is evident that the author writes from the heart and has made an invaluable and timely contribution that benefits scholars, mental health practitioners and the consumers of mental health services."

—Yegan Pillay Ph.D., P.C.C.-S

"Milt has a unique ability to describe the experience of hallucinations and delusions in a way that helps family, friends and professionals better understand, empathize and respect this condition."

—Diane Pfaff, LISW

"In this book Milt provides valuable insight and practical guidance to those who experience psychosis and delusional states and to professionals, family members and others who seek to provide help and support- an important contribution to the field."

—Steven G. Stone, Executive Director
Mental Health and Recovery Board of Ashland County

"This important work by mental health expert, Milt Greek, is a must read for those with mental illness embarking on their recovery journey and the people who love them. Through the sharing of personal stories involving psychosis, we are reminded of the vast differences that exist from one person's experience of mental illness to another. It behooves us all to learn from these experiences so we can better advocate for a system of care that meets the needs of everyone along the spectrum if or when they need it."

—NAMI Ohio

"Offering the reader an excellent overview of treatment methods (even tackling the medication vs. non-medication debate), a wealth of resources like none other (for those with lived experience and for families), and a compendium of "tools" for the practitioner and non-practitioner alike, Greek provides a truly balanced, distinctly non-agenda-driven book that is a must for all with an interest in the topic."

—Lois Oppenheim, Ph.D.

"Milt has demystified the experience of psychosis into understandable concepts to help engage clients and families while they are navigating through this process... I found it refreshing how Milt uses examples of real life people who have been able to use adversity as a gift; to find positive meaning and growth from their life as a result of their psychosis."

—Lisa Adler Bacon, MS PCC-S, LSW

"Milt Greek's most recent book, *Delusion, Meanings, and Transformation,* goes much more deeply into the topics covered in his initial book, rendering deeper understandings and weaving in approaches to treatment of psychosis that have developed in recent years. Milt draws the reader in as he interweaves his personal story, the stories of some 'fellow travelers' and multiple approaches to treatment...A very challenging book that could spark interest in adopting and integrating this 'Toolkit Approach' using those tools most helpful to each person on the road to recovery from psychosis."

—Rosemary Triggs Hayes MS, CSC, PC
Vice-Chair, Hopewell Health Care Center Board

Delusions, Meaning and Transformation

Milt Greek

Delusions, Meaning and Transformation

By Milt Greek

Copyright © 2014 Milt Greek
All rights reserved.

Cover Art "Ascend" Copyright 2014 by Karen Renee, used with permission. The author wishes to express his appreciation to Karen Renee for agreeing to allow her art to be used for this handbook.

Important Disclaimer

This book is intended for general educational purposes only. It does not substitute for individual medical advice from your doctor or legal advice from your lawyer. Please consult your doctor or lawyer for advice on your individual situation.

082914

TABLE OF CONTENTS

TABLE OF CONTENTS 1

PREFACE 5

ACKNOWLEDGEMENTS 7

MEANING AND PSYCHOSIS IN DAILY LIFE 11
   Psychosis and the personal world 13
   Ourselves 14
      Personality as a cluster of deeply-held emotions 14
      Persona and shadow 23
      Conscious and unconscious awareness 26
      Imagination 29
   The personal world 32
      Projection of the personal world self over images of the larger world 32
      Families and individual disharmony 39
      Communities and disharmony 44
      Past traumas and shadow elements 47
      Cultural scripts, icons and mythic stories 48
      World conditions and crises 49
   Some common features of psychosis 51
      Synchronicity 51
      Accurate intuitions 58
      Symbolic beliefs 61
      Coincidence and meaning 65
   Psychosis as an unrecognized vision quest 68
      Vision quests, shamanism and remarkable events in altered states 68

    Some people who experience psychosis as vision quest prone 70
    Hypothetical relationship between vision quests and psychosis 72
    Additional theoretical construct from spirituality 74

SPIRITUAL JOURNEYS 79

  Haley 82
    From addiction and nihilism to deliverance and renewal 82
    Personal world 82
    Psychosis 86
    Post-psychosis 93
  Mike 95
    Discovering sacred feminine mysteries 95
    Personal world 96
    Psychosis 102
    Post-psychosis 107
  Will 111
    Precognition leads into "delusional" religion 111
    Personal world 112
    Psychosis 116
    Post-psychosis 123
  John 126
    Self-discovery as a mystical artist 126
    Personal world 127
    Psychosis 128
    Post-psychosis 141
  Theresa 145
    From isolation to a loving family 145
    Personal world 146
    Psychosis 150
    Post-psychosis 160
  Summary observations about the spiritual journeys ... 167

A COMBINED TOOLKIT APPROACH TO PSYCHOSIS 175

The medication debate 175
Building effective treatment 179
Details of the combined toolkit approach 182
Treatment protocol to move from psychosis to
stabilization 184
    Initial work 184
    Web of life maps 191
    Beginning transformation, stabilization and recovery
    202
    Moving into stability and post-psychosis 207
Additional aspects of care 212
    Building working relationships 212
    Improving self-care 215
    Approaches to healing trauma 216
    Resources for the family 218
    Advocacy for the person 219
    Resources for the person 221
Other tools 222
Counseling and issues with counselors 223
Approaches other than the toolkit 225
Non-medical approaches 226
Witnessing the spiritual journeys of people sharing a web
of life 227

APPENDIX A COMPARISON OF TOOLS IN COMBINED TOOLKIT 231

Central aspects of toolkit 231
Relationship models 232
Self-care 235
Adopting different approaches based on individual
circumstances 235
Re-creating the person's web of life 237
Healing trauma 237
Resources for the family and the person 239
Note on psychological theories 242

APPENDIX B ADAPTING THE COMBINED TOOLKIT

FOR MEDIUM-TERM FACILITIES **245**

APPENDIX C POST-PSYCHOTIC SURVEYS **251**

Overview 251
Theoretical approach 253
The results of the evaluations 254
Detailed results of evaluation 259

APPENDIX D STIGMA AND BEING A SENSITIVE PERSON **261**

APPENDIX E WEBSITES OF INTEREST **271**

The medication debate 271
The combined toolkit 271
Support organizations 272
Additional websites 273

ABOUT MILT GREEK **275**

PREFACE

Thirty years ago, I was a young person in a deep crisis. My life became progressively worse, despite my own desires and attempts to make things better. As time passed, I was told that I had schizophrenia and was repeatedly hospitalized. My personal life was in shambles; my college career was in ruin, however, I alternatively saw myself as on a noble quest to save humanity or as a deeply disturbed person in the throes of a devastating spiritual crisis. My family and the medical establishment insisted that if I just took a pill, the world and I would be fine. To my personal good fortune, I began to take medication for schizophrenia and, at the same time, focused on a spiritual overhaul of my life and inner self based on insights gained during my psychosis. Everything good in my life since then was made possible by these two decisions.

Ten years ago, I began to outline a blueprint for recovery from schizophrenia based on my personal experience, as well as my experience volunteering with people in psychosis and post-psychosis. Since that time, numerous other blueprints for recovery have gained popularity, ranging from Open Dialogue to the Hearing Voices Movement to LEAP (Listen Empathize Agree Partner). I believe each of these approaches contains a piece of the puzzle as we work like blind men describing an elephant. We each know our own story, the stories of our fellow travelers and the research we have encountered.

In the story of blind men describing an elephant, each man insists that only his perception is accurate, resulting in no one being able to know the true shape of the elephant they all touch. I think we are all correct about our personal truth as we work through the many different forms of consciousness that have been lumped together as "psychosis." The intent of this new book is to begin a common ground approach that respects all of our stories and tries to blend the many tools created for working with people like me into a common, multifaceted approach. Part of this attempt includes the review of the life journeys of five post-psychotic people, explored deeply in the second passage. These stories are largely drawn from the results of post-psychotic surveys reviewed in Appendix C.

It can be very difficult in this highly impersonal technological age to speak from the heart. Even so, it is crucial that I acknowledge that everything I have in my life has been made possible by people like the reader of these words. Were it not for people like you—friends, family members, peers, and professionals working on behalf of someone like me—I would have nothing to offer. It is the kindness and compassion that we give each other that makes our hard human world worth living in. Thank you for caring enough to want to help someone like me. I sincerely hope you can both give and receive the kindness and compassion that we all need to live and be happy.

Milt Greek

ACKNOWLEDGEMENTS

The author wishes to sincerely thank the many people who made this book possible. Crucial to this material being created were Paul Komarek, who provided proofreading and formatting; Sharon Young of Cooper Riis and Steve Stone of the Mental Health and Recovery Board of Ashland County, both of whom challenged me to go beyond the material in my first book and kindly supported this material in presentations at their organizations; and Trey Crispin, who encouraged people at Cooper Riis to consider my work and who gave me insight through providing me an introduction to Tai Chi.

In addition, I sincerely appreciate Paris Williams and Theresa's kind permission to use material from *Rethinking Madness*. The frankness and courage of Haley, Mike, Will, John and Theresa in sharing their stories is essential for understanding some of the different experiences that have been lumped together as "psychosis."

In terms of reviewing of the text, I am very indebted to Sharon Young, Yegan Pillay, Irene Mock, Paul Komarek, Steve Stone, Betsy Johnson, Lois Oppenheim, Lisa Adler Bacon, Diane Pfaff and Rosemary Triggs Hayes.

This material is composed of numerous references to the work of others, including most centrally Ron Coleman, Xavier Amador, Mary Ellen Copeland, Pat Deegan and numerous others who have developed approaches like Open Dialogue, CBT, EMDR, Re-evaluation Counseling and eCPR. Jason's Lai's willingness to share his advice on advocacy is an important addition to this material. Without all of the invaluable contributions of these people, the combine toolkit would not exist.

Finally, I wish to thank my wife, who has supplied tremendous clarity to me over the years through our ongoing conversations about this subject, as well as many other aspects of life. Her contributions to this material cannot be measured.

DELUSIONS, MEANING AND TRANSFORMATION

MEANING AND PSYCHOSIS IN DAILY LIFE

The purpose of this passage is to help the reader connect the beliefs and experiences of people in psychosis with meaning from the person's life. Personal meaning is created by the person's life and how she or he responds to this context. Most powerfully, meaning is created by our relationships.

The relationship between the person's life and the feelings expressed in psychosis can often be summed up simply. When a son in psychosis, raised by his father after a bitterly fought divorce, greets his mother for the first time in months with paranoid rage, there is an obvious connection between the feelings of the father and his son's exaggerated and delusional state. As heart-rending as an encounter like this must be for all involved, the similarity and origin of the feelings are obvious. Father angry at mother ➜ Son absorbs father's anger ➜ Son expresses anger at mother.

Simple logic can summarize the life and feelings of people, but it is important to see life as filled with slowly unfolding dramas. The life stories of individuals, our families, communities and even the larger human and natural worlds are intertwined with complex details, making simple logic the beginning clues to unlocking the meaning of events during psychosis.

Psychosis can project one's life's meaning into consciousness—mixed so thoroughly with delusion that it seems nonsense to outsiders—and give us insight. In my own case, having my deep-seated feelings and meaning projected vividly into my conscious mind made me aware of the true context of my life. Unconscious thoughts and feelings, as well as memories too painful to face, welled up. At the same time, a vision of my life and the human world free of these hardships arose, again expressed in delusions. With time, the visions I had for a better world led to changes in my life and personality that resolved and helped heal my deepest wounds.

This passage discusses the context of our lives and how meaning, often not consciously recognized, comes to the surface in the form of exaggerated and seemingly random delusions. The promise of this process is that not only that we come to a confused consciousness about our lives but we also often envision a resolution to our life's problems. We begin a quest, both delusional and personally meaningful, to make our lives and the world as a whole significantly better.

This passage will provide some of the more prominent aspects of psychosis and meaning, providing building blocks to look at a person in psychosis and make educated guesses about the meaning of her or his experiences. This will help us understand the motivation and direction of the person's spiritual journey, opening up the process to make it a collaboration to keep the person both safe and moving along on the spiritual transformation. Examples of spiritual journeys like these are included in the second passage, in which five people speak about their lives prior to, during and after psychosis.

The intention is to provide some building blocks for psychological observation but not to build a very strong theoretical structure. Meaning systems, such as Freud's and Jung's, can have merit if applied in a piecemeal fashion, but ultimately each person is unique. If you wish to know the meaning of anything to a person, it is essential to know his or her personal life and compassionately explore the person's journey as a fellow human being. That unique experience, different than mine and different than yours, is the heart and soul of the meaning we seek to discover.

PSYCHOSIS AND THE PERSONAL WORLD

To understand psychosis it is important to recognize that it often brings about a positive spiritual quest. The experience of hallucinations and other dream-like aspects of psychosis cause the person's life to be projected into his or her consciousness the way a film projector shows the content of films. Psychosis is like a waking dream in which the surrounding world is mirrored in seemingly fantastic and symbolic ways, just as a person sleeping with the TV on will often have a dream that parallels the TV program in different but clear ways.

With this projection of one's life in psychosis, the significant aspects of one's life are highlighted dramatically. Aspects that cause turmoil—ranging from personal trauma or failings to real, large world crises—are thrown into our consciousness and made unbearable by the intensity of the challenge. The psychotic experience becomes a catalyst for change that can bring forth a significantly better life for the person and those around him or her. The potential for spiritual and/or psychological growth during and after psychosis does not make it any less of a heart-rending crisis. For those outside the experience—family members, friends, professionals and peers—psychosis is a mysterious and terrifying event which makes the person irrational and a threat to well-being and life itself.

To help understand a person's psychosis, find ways to communicate, calm and stabilize the person, and bring the psychosis to resolution, I will look at common aspects of life that, when projected into psychosis, becomes the basis for hallucinations and delusions. I will set aside the discussion of psychosis to look at elements of our lives as vulnerable and imperfect people living in the emotionally thick context of family and community webs of life.

OURSELVES

Personality as a cluster of deeply-held emotions

Western culture as I experience it is insistent on the pretense of paying attention to each other's emotions. In my work life, I meet coworkers on the elevator and elsewhere and out of politeness ask them how they are. According to the rules of our culture, they are supposed to say, "Good" or "Fine" or complain about having to work and ask how I am. We then discuss the weather, sports or some other topic that is meant to divert our attention from each other as real people with deeply powerful stories, traumas, hardships and hopes for a better life.

Only when tragedy strikes and coworkers discretely inform each other that a workmate will not be in because someone close to them is gravely ill or has passed on is it acceptable for someone to publically express sorrow, regret, loss or other vulnerable emotions. Friendships among workers are exceptions, where people tentatively throw off the façade of perfect lives with perfect families and begin to express our hopes, dreams, challenges and sorrows that successful, well-adjusted people are supposed to have either attained or overcome. Those who violate these norms with public expressions of emotions (other than anger and indignation at poorly done work) are generally avoided as needy and weak individuals who make us uncomfortable with their violation of our culture's agreed-upon rules that we will ignore each other's emotional life.

Many of us learn to ignore emotions or lack the details needed to understand why people feel as they do. By habitually ignoring emotions, it is common to be, as I was, largely blind to the emotional content of conversations. Feelings become unconscious the way that telephone poles along roads become unconscious. We know they are there but only notice them when something brings them to our attention. In learning to see feelings, it helps to purposefully focus on voice tone, facial expressions, the look of the eyes and body language and to get to know the story of people's lives. We then get a clear picture of the person. In doing so, the hidden world of feelings can be seen as the center of our lives and personalities.

As young children grow older, different emotional affinities can be seen with different children. Some children are mechanically-inclined, working with models, bikes and motors; others enjoy drawing, painting and poetry; a third group love sports and physical activity; a fourth set of children may be academic in nature, loving to read and doing well in their studies. Many children are combinations of these and other affinities. As children grow older, many become interested in partying with alcohol, sex and possibly drugs while others naturally fit into a more religious mode that emphasizes sobriety and chastity. Likewise, as young adults, some people are focused primarily on careers of making money while others go into social work and charitable activities as expressions of their altruistic natures.

Temperaments are another deeply held part of personality. Some people are joking in nature, some are angry, some melancholy, some anxious, while others are often carefree and happy-go-lucky. Most people have a small set of moods that dominate their lives as they cycle through these different moods. Significantly, our own moods are very important in determining what we pay attention to and how we react to the personal world around us, but we are oftentimes ignorant that these few, dominating moods are constructing our personal reality by shaping our actions and reactions to others.

In addition to these internal qualities, our personal history, the traumas we endure and the times we are protected from the consequences of our actions play crucial roles in shaping how we relate to our web of life. Long-term pressure to conform to something that goes against our inner nature can also be similar to trauma. Trauma creates fear, anger, depression and separating off from the world around us. It usually also creates negative habits which distract us from the trauma, including addictions. At the same time, growing up without facing the consequences of our actions can create personalities who blithely ignore the harm we do and trigger conflict because we lack regard for others.

Our relationships in our personal world become embedded in our life history, with harmony and disharmony between our affinities and temperaments and the people around us. Trauma, pressure to conform and protection from natural consequences become embedded in different combinations in these relationships, creating powerful emotional substructures in our web of life. As young people grow older, those who have experienced a lot of trauma will usually become very rebellious and react against the affinities and teachings of people they associate the trauma with.

These deeply held, long lasting emotions and emotional cycles are the substructure that words, events and consciousness are aimed at expressing. Like bridge pylons sunk deep into the riverbed, the emotional structures of personality are the foundation for how people act and interact. When one coworker is habitually anxious and pessimistic about every new work initiative and another is notorious for a bad temper and impatience with coworkers, it is obvious that these emotional habits are expressing deeply held feelings. These emotions, repeatedly expressed on a near-daily basis, have very little to do with the topic my coworkers are talking about. Rather, these are feelings coming up from their personal lives that they disguise—even to themselves—as about something else.

In many ways it is the world close to us—our personal world—that is central to who we are. I might, as I did during my psychosis, argue loudly with classmates about the direction the outside world should go in, while many sit out the arguments. Despite our different viewpoints, those of us who spent our days arguing had many emotions in common, while those who sat out the arguments had emotions different from us. The outer world issues of politics, religion and so forth were largely covers for us to vent our inner anger. Despite our differing worldviews, our temperaments were largely the same.

By discounting larger world attachments, we can look at relationships as made up of strong affinities and aversions. In these personal world relationships—our web of life—we develop emotional cycles with those around us, spiraling over the years, for better and worse, into our young adulthood. These undercurrents form our attachments and cement relationships with strong sentiments, habits and expectations about each.

Seeing how people react to emotional expression, what emotions are shared and who is allowed to express different emotions helps contextual the emotions. A father may be allowed to express anger, but his children cannot. An older brother may be able to criticize younger siblings, but not vice versa. A child with a wry and clever sense of humor may be welcomed as a source of joy or condemned as disrespectful. Who is allowed to express what emotions are statements about power in relationships and shape the inner emotional world of all involved.

Looking at what feelings is directed at who is central to understanding emotional undercurrents. For example, it is common for high prestige children to vent their anger onto lower status children. The lower status children, who are the scapegoats of their school-age community, will often internalize these emotions and live out self-destructive patterns in their early adulthood. The same is common with victims of childhood abuse.

Once patterns like these are instilled, young adults will have learned where to direct their negative and positive feelings in ways that either fit into the mold of their family and community cultures or that are purposeful and defiant choices in the opposite direction. In learning these emotional directions and life stories, it is possible to begin seeing underlying emotional structures and cycles in relationships.

In very close relationships, emotions are shared like an unconscious sixth sense. After years of living together, a family and community's emotional roles and cycles have largely been worked out. The pillars of the community and the golden children are given prestige and consideration, while the malcontents and eccentrics are used as scapegoats to vent unhappiness. The dominant people in the family are given deference, and are protected from criticism, while the black sheep and wayward children are sharply rebuked for their own good. People will know their roles well, reacting to each other out of habit and repeating cycles in their relationships. In doing so, the outer world artifice that is expressed in habits of words and actions is the topcoat of underlying emotions.

One example of cycles is found in abusive relationships, which are disturbingly common in our communities, especially in the lives of young women. In these relationships, the abuser commonly experiences a buildup of stress from outside problems, insults, or losses. The abuser will then strike out at the victim, who is seen as triggering and deserving the abuse. The abuse will sometimes go unreported but sometimes will be witnessed or reacted against by the victim seeking outsiders to intervene. At this point, the abuser often expresses a form of regret, saying that if the victim had only not done a certain act that everything would have been fine. After some drama, the victim will give into the abuser and the relationship cycle will begin again.

Over time, the friends and family of the victim will seek to help the victim. However, in many cases the victim feels love and dependency towards the abuser and will cut off relationships with others who want to intervene on her behalf. At the same time, others will break off relationships with the couple.

As the couple becomes more isolated from healthy people, the victim begins to accept the rationalizations of the abuser within her own thinking. If she were to only not do certain things, everything would work out. However, since the abuser is really displacing feelings of anger from other situations, the abuse continues until the victim reaches a breaking point and angrily rejects the abuser once and for all.

In another common cycle, people with substance abuse problems will cycle into greater and greater amounts of drug and alcohol use, becoming increasingly dysfunctional, harming relationships and acting erratically. After months or even years of growing dependency, a crisis will ensue, such as an injury, the end of a romantic relationship or some other meaningful loss, and the addicted person will resolve to sober up. For a period of time, ranging from a few weeks to a few years, he or she will live a more sober life. At a certain point, sometimes during a time where the person's life may seem to be finally coming together or during a time of crisis, she or he will backslide into initially minor amounts of drinking or drug use. Over time, the addiction issues will emerge and the cycle will once again descend into heavy use, dysfunction and unhappy relationships.

Emotional cycles like these, along with many others, commonly occur in our families and communities. Oftentimes the cycles will become set and couples will become parents, with their children learning to fit into these cycles. Along with the more notorious cycles outlined above, cycles involving relationships, work, career, finances and numerous other aspects of life occur as people and our families mature. This often leads to young people who have been greatly affected by both positive and negative family patterns that are considered by those involved to be the natural and normal way of life for most people.

As young adults leave one web of life for another, there seems to be an emotional drive akin to a homing drive, probably related to what psychologists call our attachment—our love—for our family, friends and community. Our personality's attachment to those around us will attract us as teenagers and young adults to people and things that seem familiar—that we fit in with and can relate to out of our habitual self. In doing so, our lives re-create our childhood web of life, often replaying the traumas and patterns witnessed in the families and communities we grew up in. Our adult life paths often begin as reflections of the journeys of our families and communities, sometimes despite our conscious intentions to live in very different ways. This repetition of family patterns is evident in the story of Mike in the second passage.

For long-lasting change, deeply held emotions must be altered permanently. Yet these emotions are cemented in place by years of our experience, including trauma, sorrow, loss and confusion. Deeply held emotions are usually transformed slowly, if ever, by events or changes in our web of life. Personal change and spiritual growth occurs over decades, with times of rapid change followed by long periods of adjustment making the changes real in our personal world.

Our long-term relationships are largely permanent emotional structures that are set and out of any one person's control. When a father and son are bitterly set against each other, few can alter the decades-long drama that ensues. When a parent favors one child over others, family relationships can be twisted by jealously and bitter rivalry. These relationships have trauma, hardship, challenges, dreams and aspirations embedded in them, some of which are very painful. People, especially young people, will dream of better things and will want to transcend the hardship of our lives whether or not psychosis develop.

Psychosis, with its projection of emotional undercurrents into our consciousness, creates a person who no longer finds the roles and hardships that we all endure to be bearable. To the dismay and fear of family and community, the person in psychosis begins a strange and mystifying journey to transform or leave our original web of life, believing that we are on a magical quest transforming our lives and the entire world. Beyond the risks and hardships of psychosis, our delusions and actions are disconcerting for family and community because family and community cultures are violated. In the early phase of psychosis, we no longer fit in and we eagerly anticipate a new life in a new world.

Persona and shadow

As young children we discover we are expected to show a positive exterior to the outside world. We learn to say we are "Fine" even though we may privately be sad or angry. As we mature, we learn to "put our best foot forward" and "put on a happy face," turning into adults who understand we and our families are to appear happy, competent and confident. People who share their private trials too easily are avoided for violating public cultural space for being needy. People who put on a good show are admired for their personal strength. For example, during college a roommate of mine told how a dorm mate had been fun and lively at the party; only afterwards did my roommate learn that the fun-living life of the party had just been rejected by a girl he had been very interested in. The roommate felt the other fellow was mature and strong in the face of emotional adversity.

Carl Jung, a psychoanalyst, called the public face we show the world our "Persona," or mask, which hides deeper feelings, protecting us and projecting the expected image. Personas vary from person to person—some are fun-loving jokers, some are no-nonsense businesspeople, some are intellectual observers and so forth—and also affect our consciousness. When we spend a lot of time in public circles, putting forth our persona, we tend to forget private troubles we may be going through.

For many people, the persona is closely tied to the self-image, especially if the person is focused on outer-world achievements. By spending many hours on career, or on outer world hobbies like sports, daily thoughts focus on the outer world and the persona, causing us to forget the more powerful parts of our private life. People who are successful in the outer world often lose track of our private, personal life.

The cluster of traits that people do not want to face, things that we fear about who we are, is what Jung called "The Shadow." The shadow contains our traumas, our negative qualities, our fears and other things we do not want to look at. The persona put forward can often be an opposite of the shadow as an attempt to hide these qualities. For example, someone who felt inferior to others as a child may become competitive with others and develop into an "aggressive athlete" or a "know-it-all," attempting to prove to others (and mainly to ourselves) that she or he is superior, not inferior. People who use their homes and families as dumping grounds for their frustrations may be smooth and charming to outsiders. The conscientious church mother who devotes long hours to community service may berate her children as inadequate and ungrateful; the charming and easy-going coworker may go home and scream at his wife because of a moment where he felt insulted by a boss. When someone shows a public face that is the opposite of her or his private self, denial causes the person to hide the painful private issues in his or her shadow.

In daily life, many aspects of the emotional structures that underlie our lives are placed into the shadows of individuals, families and communities. Our consciousness naturally looks outward at the more pleasant parts of our lives in the persona and turns away from the shadows elements, making these important but unhappy parts of our lives largely unconscious.

Seeing our shadow is emotionally painful. We become aware of things about ourselves we do not like and recall trauma that we do not want to face. When our shadow aspects are touched on we feel pain; when someone brings them to our attention people often react with indignation and anger. We attempt to maintain denial about the things we don't want to face, seeking to drive away or silence the person who is forcing us to face up to our negative qualities and unhappy memories. When elements of the collective shadow—aspects shared by our community or society—are brought to public view, gatekeepers of public consciousness quickly work to attack and silence the people bringing these negative aspects to light. For a patriot of any country, it is intolerable to have the country's negative qualities brought to public view and those who do so are maligned as disloyal and a threat to the country's welfare. Those in the dominant religion of a society will condemn those who question its tenets as "ungodly" and "facing God's wrath," regardless of the actual characters of the people involved.

In psychosis, the shadow cannot be avoided. The projection of our lives into our hallucinations and delusions means that our personal and collective shadow will be dramatically brought to our consciousness in highly metaphorical events, sometimes with encounters with religious figures like Jesus, angels and saints. As time goes on, these projections tell us a story that is a commentary on our lives and has themes that bring the shadow elements to light. In highly symbolic and dramatic terms we face personal, family, community, national and international problems that are frequently swept under the rug. We feel a need to explore the world deeply and resolve the problems we are becoming aware of.

At the painful time when we encounter the shadow within us and begin to explore the unconscious world people seek to deny, we begin to have insights about the connections permeating our life history and personal world. Jung pointed out that being able to face the shadow was the gateway to the unconscious, allowing us insights into part of ourselves and others that are normally kept hidden. We begin to understand why people around us react with the emotions they do and how previously unrecognized events have created the social and emotional world around us.

As we misinterpret personal symbolic events as literal events with universal meaning, we link these beliefs with our real life, giving them weight and importance. When we believe that Jesus or an angel has given us a message about something that needs changed, we may inflate the scope of the message away from our personal world into a worldwide problem, but our personal issues are seen as one example of this worldwide problem. By trying to magically solve the world's problems, we are also trying to solve our real-life challenges that our encounter with our shadow has brought to light.

Conscious and unconscious awareness

Understanding people who enter psychosis requires recognizing that we are facing previously unconscious aspects of our lives. While people vary in how much of our lives are not really consciously recognized, seeing psychosis as containing knowledge new to us mixed with misperception and random events is important in understanding our initial excitement in "discovering new truths." For most of us, our conscious mind focuses on day-to-day living and thoughts, going through phases as our moods and energy level change. Being conscious of our personal world and ourselves parallel what physiologists call voluntary motions like moving an arm to pick up a coffee cup or using our arms and legs to drive a car. If less tangible aspects of our lives, such as the feelings and patterns in relationships around us are conscious, we can seek to change and improve with them focused effort.

In my experience, our conscious mind not only focuses our attention and allows us to carry out tasks; it also acts as a gatekeeper to keep out distracting and unacceptable thoughts that might slip in from our shadow. In psychosis, the central inner voice that we equate with who we are breaks down and our minds are filled with voices that say things, such as racist slurs or obscenities, which our conscious mind would not normally allow. The central voice is not only the speaker of our thoughts but also the moderator for what thoughts are allowed to be said or focused on.

Aspects of our lives that we are not conscious of parallel what are called involuntary motions, such as our heart beating and our lungs breathing. We cannot control these very well and, in these examples, we cannot live if we stop them altogether. Unconscious parts of our emotional and personal world can be very difficult to alter or control, especially when they are part of patterns with people around us. Things that are hidden by our shadows—such as traumas, negative traits and desires that are frightening to admit having—create emotional impulses separate from conscious thought and affect our lives without our awareness or control. If someone with a strong shadow does happen to think of these impulses, the recognition is often quickly forgotten as a way to avoid the pain of facing the shadow. People in psychosis can become aware of these unconscious patterns, often inflating our personal world into universal scenarios.

Unconscious aspects of life frequently involve the effect of people's deeply held emotions on our lives. A person with unresolved anger may frequently bring up hot button issues like politics and religion with people different from her or him, frequently arguing with people and being thought of as a difficult person. Another person may have experienced painful unresolved loss and feels that pain when she or he is resting. Rather than experience the pain, the person may fill his or her life with activity, becoming a workaholic or activist, to distract her or him from the pain that wells up when not doing something. In another, common, example, a child or young adult may have a beloved family member die or have a very painful romance and after that sabotage promising relationships to avoid the risk of another heartbreaking loss.

Our unconscious impulses, though able to sense feelings, are unable to plan or recognize the consequences of our actions. This was observed by Sigmund Freud, who saw the Id as powerful unconscious impulses that does not understand the outside world. A person whose buried anger makes them unconsciously argumentative with those around him or her will drive away many people but will be unable to consciously recognize the pattern or face the anger buried in her or his shadow. Likewise, those fleeing inner pain by becoming workaholics or avoiding intimacy and committed relationships may not consciously recognize the source of their behavior. Most of the content of our shadows and the memories behind them are not malevolent; instead the shadow often contains painful, unhealed memories and feelings that we try to throw into the back of our emotional closet, only to have our lives driven by these forgotten hardships. In psychosis, these unconscious patterns within and around us are projected into our delusional consciousness in symbolic, meaningful hallucinations and beliefs, causing us to face our shadows in stark and dramatic ways.

Facing our shadows is painful, but, as my wife eloquently put it, "The gift of consciousness is control of our lives." By facing our shadow and seeing how our unconscious feelings and patterns—whether they are abusive towards others, makes us the victims of others, or somehow hides traumas and desires we do not wish to face—we have the potential to gain control of our choices and our lives, stopping patterns which harm us and gaining insight into making our lives and those around us better, healthier and happier.

Imagination

Though discounted in our secular worldviews, recognizing the role of imagination and different perspectives on it is central to understanding those in psychosis. In the modern, secular world, imagination is viewed as an inner experience with little or no consequences. Daydreams, fantasies, memories, inner dialogues and other aspects of our imaginations are considered to have no consequences unless acted on. Forms of shared imagination, such as computer and video games, fiction in media and so forth are of little importance from a secular viewpoint.

Inner imagination and the imagination shared with others often contains raw, vulnerable, conflicting and fleeting emotions and symbolic fantasies which express feelings we do not want show the world and are often expressions of inners fears, anger, resentments and unmet desires. In modern times, imagination is used to vent our fears and frustrations, resulting in many movies, shows and games that are filled with negative emotions. Our fantasies are also expressed in media that show remarkably handsome people with very expensive homes in high-cost cities who are, somehow, easy for us to identify with. From a secular viewpoint, our modern world's fascination with shared imagination—whether it is in scandalous behavior in so-called reality shows, graphic violence in action-adventure movies or in the wealth of people's homes—is harmless and has no consequences. With this perspective, our imaginations are set free to express our inner feelings without any sense of limits.

From a religious point of view, what we think about is important because it can lead to negative behavior. If we allow thoughts that could lead to temptations to hold sway, we are likely to fail in the tests of our lives. For religious thinkers and activists, it is a common statement that "Thought is the most important aspect of spiritual life" because what we think leads to what we do. Dwelling on sexual thoughts, for example, can lead to promiscuity and a myriad of problems when uncontrolled sexuality has unintended consequences. Praying regularly and seeking to regulate one's inner thinking and feelings is part of a devotional life, providing a path to overcome the challenges of the material world.

For some religions, especially Eastern religions, there is extensive practice of meditation and chanting aimed at "churning our minds" into the proper state to pursue a religious life. Meditation is not "staring at one's navel," but rather mental and emotional exercises aimed at transforming our inner spirit to be one with the sacred aspects of the universe. Western religions also advocate prayer and devotion to reconcile our spirits to the will of the Deity. By doing so the temptations of Earthly life can be overcome and our souls made ready to meet the Deity in the afterlife.

From a mystical viewpoint, the inner world of thought, desire and imagination is more than something to be transformed to conform to the sacred. Mysticism sees the mind as a launching pad for events. Our imaginations are gateways to our futures, bringing complementary people and events into our lives and allowing the spiritual world to manifest our thoughts and desires. "Be careful what you wish for" is not a trivial statement to a mystical person—it is a warning that our inner thoughts and desires take form in our lives whether we intend them to or not.

These different perspectives on imagination are essential to understanding the feelings of someone who is psychotic. In the modern world, many people grow up with a secular view of imagination and have little practice in controlling our inner thoughts and feelings. As psychosis projects our life into seemingly real events, many people experiencing psychosis go from thinking of imagination as of no importance to seeing it in an extremely exaggerated mystical viewpoint. From this viewpoint, thoughts and feelings are constantly manifesting in reality around us. All forms of media such as television and internet can bring about changes in reality through the spiritual energy they emit. As real life events are reflected in ongoing hallucinations and delusions, as reported in the stories of Haley and Will, we believe we have concrete proof that mind over matter is a constant part of life.

With this new perspective on imagination, our habits of thinking, feeling, fantasy and daydreams take on a new light. No longer are they insignificant past times—they are frequently seen as the key determination of our fate and that of the larger world. Our imagination can easily become confused with reality, first by seeing the connections between our inner and outer world, then in believing that the metaphors of our imaginary world have some real universal meaning and finally by believing these metaphors are literal, actual realities that are independent of our existence. If our imagination prior to psychosis was used to imagine vampires and aliens in fantasy, our psychosis will seem populated with real life vampires and aliens; if we frequently spoke with Jesus in prayer prior to psychosis, we will then walk with and possibly become Jesus during our psychosis.

THE PERSONAL WORLD

Projection of the personal world self over images of the larger world

When we think of the human world, we tend to think of the world in terms of images we have seen in the media, rather than our personal world. Our modern culture attracts our attention away from our here and now personal world and towards the outside world. However, it can be very difficult to know what the outside world is really like. This is true not only for things outside our personal space, but also for things that are in the past or the future. To know about the world outside our here and now we must rely on portals such as television, radio, the internet and email.

People tend to be attracted to specific portals to the outside world, such as particular news channels or websites, which are familiar and help confirm one's view of things over conflicting views, especially when challenged by views that bring the shadow to consciousness. For example, a businessperson making money through natural gas and oil will be attracted to media sources that reject climate change as being caused by human activity; a person from a military family will avoid media sources that cause him or her to question the righteousness of their county's wars. On the other hand, people are attracted to news that shows the negative (shadow) aspects of those they consider rivals or enemies.

Despite our modern focus on the outside world, the personal world is the primary motivator for many people. Many people in our personal world may use the outside world to attempt to manipulate the personal world, while remaining motivated by the personal world. For example, people who are "know-it-alls," people who incessantly argue about politics and religious people who proselytize others often claim special knowledge and authority about the outside world. They often see themselves in grandiose terms as offering insight about the larger world to help those around them, but they are often motivated by unhealed pain that makes them angry and desiring to control conversation and people.

It is noteworthy that a person's spiritual connection (which is actually here and now) can create a miraculously strong will, allowing people who tap into it to suddenly overcome powerful addictions and negative behavior. At the same time, people can claim authority over this powerful connection by insisting that they know the mind and will of the Deity, thereby allowing them to control vulnerable others. The power given by one's connection to the spiritual world and the power-over-others that comes from claiming special authority over that connection figure strongly in the journey of Haley that is told in the second passage.

One of the most important realizations about the outside world is that most beliefs about it are not refutable. For example, I am fairly certain that the Russian city of Moscow exists, but if someone were to insist it did not I would have a very hard time proving it does. As we move farther and farther away from the here and now there is less and less certainty. Because of this, the outside world and everything that is not in the here and now is prone to our projecting onto it whatever beliefs we desire.

During psychosis, the larger world is often a metaphor for personal world, just as many people not in psychosis use the outside world to project their beliefs. With those of us who experience psychosis, the larger world is often synonymous with our personal world, with the delusions that are exaggerated references to our own life taken as literal, outer world realities. For example, the common belief in psychosis that the "end of the world" is approaching often represents the unconscious awareness that our personal dysfunction and hardships are leading to the collapse of our personal world. In a happier overlaying of the larger world with the personal world, the journey of Theresa in seeking to save the larger world led her to save her personal world.

People in psychosis are often motivated by not here now beliefs, which can be very impractical for anyone. In someone who is in psychosis this can sometimes be very dangerous. Understanding the importance of these beliefs and connecting them to the real life of the person can aid in working with the person and keeping her or him calm and safe. For example, when a person in psychosis has a plan to save the world, the question to ask is "In what way is this plan symbolically or actually related to saving her or his personal web of life?"

To understand underlying connections in a person's not here now beliefs, it is helpful to look at the emotions expressed by the beliefs, the person expressing them, the other people around them and the direction of the emotion. For example, beliefs that say from one person to another that "You are condemned" represents anger from the person towards the other and are aimed at controlling the other person. Such anger often is a reaction from the fears of the shadow, so the anger can be reversed to see the inner fears of the person who is sending it out. For example, if someone has overcome a drug addiction and has deep-seated fears of backsliding into the addiction again, he or she may lecture about the evils of drugs and the wicked souls of those using them as a means to keep distance from the drug use she or he fears falling back into. This reaction-formation of personality development was noted by Sigmund Freud and is found in the stories of Haley, Mike, and Theresa in the second passage.

Another common set of beliefs in psychosis is summed up by "I am condemned," such as when a person believes that she or her are condemned by god, an evil being doomed for punishment, the worst soul in the universe and so forth. This self-loathing is anger from the person back towards his or her self. This emotion usually originates from others and is often linked to a painful rejection by someone close to her or him, sometimes in the past, sometimes recently and oftentimes both. At the same time, this self-loathing can also indicate a real life moral dilemma or severe character flaw that the person wants to overcome but cannot. In the same way, people in psychosis may hurt themselves, which is a terrifying acting out of the anger aimed at themselves. An example of rejection, without a severe character flaw, causing a sense of self-loathing leading to a suicide attempt is in the journey of John. In another example, the internal character issues that Mike was concerned about led to hallucinations that made him believe he was condemned.

When we look at beliefs about the outside world that seem nonsensical, but are very important to the person in psychosis, it is helpful to ask questions to connect real life information to symbolic delusions.

- How do the emotions of the delusion parallel emotions from real life?
- What would be the effect if these emotions and beliefs were respected in the person's web of life?

- What would a psychologically healthy person be seeking?
- What are unique qualities of the person in psychosis's personality?
- How do the delusions, themes and events represent an unfolding of the person's inner self?

If we connect the delusions and the emotions they express to the person's real life context, we can seek to remedy the personal issues by changing the web of life around the person. As our real life issues improve, the delusions that express those issues will improve and trust is built between the person and the people trying to help.

Speech is also like the outside world in that speaking can often feel very important but words alone often have few consequences. Speech should be looked at like outer world beliefs with attention to the emotions expressed and the direction of the emotions. Like things that are not here now, conversation with family and friends has few meaningful consequences unless the person violates a web of life consensus rule. As a result, people develop habitual ways of speaking that expresses inner emotions. For example, a person who tends to argue with just about everyone about just about everything will tend to have free-floating anger from unresolved hurt and conflict. People who express fears of a conspiracy of secret, powerful cadres often are experiencing a deep sense of helplessness in their own lives.

In a particularly useful example, I knew two impoverished white sisters, one of whom was the single mother of an interracial child, who talked about a city where people were known to "step into other worlds," disappearing from the street and leaving this world. One sister expressed a strong desire to go to the city and try to step into another world.

If the sisters had said this in a psychiatrist's office, they would have been labeled delusional. However, by looking at their life situation, the emotions and desires come from obvious sources. The two impoverished sisters had New Age mystical beliefs in very religiously conservative and racist part of the rural south. They were constantly asked by people they met what church they went to and they felt so frightened of revealing their New Age beliefs that they told people the New Age books on their bookshelves were science fiction. They feared for themselves and the interracial child of one of the sisters, lacked community support, and were too poor to find a way to move.

As time went by, the sisters did find a way to move to a city in the north where there was less racial and religious oppression and they were closer to their family. They found work and began new lives with much less community stress. After this, the sisters stopped talking about cities where people stepped into other worlds because they had stepped into a better world, just as their "delusional" belief had envisioned. To some depth psychologists, the purpose of the belief may have been more than simply an expression of the seemingly delusional solution; it may have been way to unconsciously set into motion the events that allowed them to leave behind an oppressive personal world and move to a better, more supportive personal world.

Families and individual disharmony

In the face-to-face personal world, it is difficult to measure the degree of family dysfunction to know the normal range of unhappiness, conflict and disharmony. In many communities, some families seek a public competition, attempting to show in the community's public space that their family is more successful, happier and better adjusted than others. These competitions are often based on what that individual tends to value. Those who fit into a traditional religious mold may talk about their service to their local church; people oriented towards making money will discuss their successful careers and material wealth; individuals focused on intellectual pursuits will speak of the prestigious universities and degrees that they have attended and attained.

Just as people have personas and shadows, families have a face they try to show the world and a private life they seek to hide. Communities with a competition for prestige also have gossip mills that thrive on the troubles and scandals exposed when family shadows come into view. This allays the fears of those who look out onto the personas that people put forward and worry that their family's private dramas and dysfunction are much worse than the average family.

In looking at families and psychosis, seeing families as tightly bound sets of emotional patterns linking people to a collective fate is essential. Family life affects a person in psychosis most strongly by the forms of disharmony and trauma within it. Family disharmony can be well within the normal range and still be part of the content of delusions of a person in psychosis. Looking at different levels of disharmony provides examples of how family content can be mirrored in the beliefs and experiences of people in psychosis.

In one example, a family with three generations of men who chose engineering as careers shared with offspring who are artistic shows an intergenerational family pattern. In the first family, the father and two sons become engineers, while a daughter is drawn towards art, including painting, drawing, pottery and music. As the daughter matured, she felt distinctively different from the mechanical and money-oriented family culture. As an adult, she moved away from the family, living in a bohemian community and marrying a man with little interest in making money. Meanwhile, one of her engineer brothers married and largely repeated the family culture. As this second-generation family matured, one son repeated his family's interest and love of engineering, while another son was much more interested in music and art. The artistic son struggled with feeling very different from his family and, like his aunt, in adulthood moved into a bohemian, artistic community and married an artistic woman matching his own inclinations.

This intergenerational story of family culture and disharmony, existing without psychosis, tells of people who are distinctly different than each other and of the struggle that the person who does not fit in feels to find his or her own place in life. While not a story involving objective measures of trauma, the sense of difference within the family could easily create a tension that could be a source of content for a person in psychosis. As in the journey recounted by John, the disharmony between the family identity and the individual's inner self creates a tension within the person that is reflected in the experiences during psychosis.

In an example from a family with more dysfunction, the story of Mike involves a family with generations of anger and abuse, marked by Mike's adoption of pacifism despite a family and community culture at odds with the philosophy. Given the history of conflict within the family, the choice of the child to become a pacifist is a clear reaction to the family culture. As told in this journey, when Mike had a crisis where he faced challenges to his adopted philosophy, he developed psychosis dramatically highlighting both his struggle and his family's history, making the family content central to the content of his psychosis. The psychosis both highlighted his personal and family life and provided a dramatic playing out of his inner desire to escape his family patterns of conflict. As a result, the psychosis was a powerful catalyst for personal and spiritual growth.

Family content can also be seen where children express the feelings of parents and/or others in exaggerated form. In one case, I received a series of emails from a father whose son was in psychosis and living with the father. The parents were divorced and the mother lived several hours away. The father told me how the mother had come to visit the psychotic son during a tense situation and the son had flown into panicked rage at his mother, screaming at her to not invade his personal space. This heart-rending situation must have been very painful for all of the family members.

After the emails describing this, the father mentioned that he and the mother of his child had divorced when the son was eight or so and the parents had spent years in court seeking to gain custody of the child. The father had gained custody, so the son had grown up with the father and had a distant relationship with his mom. Looking at family content and psychosis, part of the son's rage at the mother is an expression of the father's anger at the mother. It is far too simplistic to say the son is simply parroting the father's feelings; rather, understanding the family history and the perspective of the son, both in his psychotic beliefs and in the real-life events that feed them, is central to finding some healing in this very painful family situation.

Family dynamics, as well as family history, can play a very important role with people who are mentally ill. In a widely circulated story in the mentally ill subculture after the tragedy at Sandy Hook, a mother described how her mentally ill but genius son would fly into rages when having to conform to authority. In the example she told, her thirteen-year-old son was enrolled in a school that required him to wear khaki or black pants but not navy blue pants. One morning the son tried to go to school in navy blue pants and when told he could not, insisted his pants were black. As the mother tried to get him to conform, he flew into a violent rage and the mom drove him to a mental hospital where he was put under lock and key.

From the perspective of a parent, it is easy to understand losing patience with a child who reacts with anger frequently; this is a natural response. Given the description here it appears that the child with authority issues has been placed in a military or quasi-military academy, possibly as a result of being expelled from his normal school. This response, which is a common one, may actually be setting up the child for failure. Questions which point to the child's unique needs include "Why is a child with authority issues going to a school with a much more stringent dress code than most?" and "Why is a 13 year old being asked to tell the difference between navy blue and black when many adults cannot?" Recognizing through these questions the likelihood that the child's symptoms are being worsened by the environment indicates that the decision to send the child with authority issues to a strict school may be causing more conflict with authority, actually worsening the child's behavior. While it is certainly natural to lose patience with someone who reacts angrily most of the time, it is possible that the family dynamics and choices are working against the best interests of everyone involved.

In an example from a family with significant levels of dysfunction and trauma, a mother of an adult son in psychosis discussed with me her son's belief that he had been sexually abused by his father. As the conversation continued, the mom indicated that she and the father were divorced and that the father was a narcissist who was severely emotionally abusive and alcoholic. The childhood of her children had been marked by her and her children being victimized by this abuse and the father remained unchanged. She was certain, however, that the father had not actually molested their son.

In looking at this, the sexual abuse, even if not true, is an expression of emotional abuse suffered by the son and the rest of his family. One approach to this is to use Xavier Amador's LEAP (Listen, Empathize, Agree (and agree to disagree) and Partner) technique. The mother can listen to her son's distressing statements, fully hearing what he is saying and empathizing with him, saying his feelings must be extremely painful. She can agree that the father was emotionally abusive and explain that she cannot confirm that the son was sexually abused, but they can come to common ground. Since his father was and is abusive, she will work with the son to create a safe personal space where the father will not be allowed and she will work to gain allies with the treatment team to expand this safe space to include the rest of the family outside the father.

In looking at this solution, we may have found the purpose of the beliefs held by the son. By saying that the father is sexually abusive, the son, if believed, would create a situation where the father would likely be separated from the rest of the family, allowing the family to have sanctuary away from their abuser. The prospect of a safe space without the father present and the possibility of expanding this space to include more members of the family could easily aid in calming the son and helping him stabilize.

Communities and disharmony

As noted previously with the two sisters and stress from their community, disharmony between individuals and families with the surrounding community can affect the content of "delusional" or metaphorical beliefs. Looking at the real life problems expressed in these beliefs and finding mundane solutions can help alleviate the disharmony that fuels the beliefs and the need to act on them. The sisters, by moving from a repressive community to a community more accepting of their beliefs and the race of their child and a stronger support system, the metaphorical beliefs that they could go to a city and "step into another world" were made real, much to the benefit of their family.

Similar examples in the area of delusional beliefs and religion are found in the journeys of Mike and John described in the second passage. In the first case, Mike grew up in a hostile Christian community where he was constantly told that he was condemned because he "did not accept Christ as his savior"—which Mike saw as actually meaning that he conform to the community's rejection of the theory of evolution and to practices of sexism and racial intolerance. When Mike experienced psychosis he had a series of religious hallucinations that convinced him he was condemned to hell. Like the example of the son who appears to absorb his father's anger at his mother, a simple observation is that during his psychosis Mike was overwhelmed by sentiments instilled by the hostile community around him.

In another case, John, a man raised in a Christian family who remained devout into his early teen years, saw himself during psychosis as Jesus and thought he was to be crucified when he was taken to mental hospital. In this case, the harmony between the family and community's view of Christianity and the young man's view of himself allowed enough similarities that he saw himself as holy and saw events as following the story of Jesus's suffering.

In both of these cases, it is important to see the details of the person's life and how they intertwine with their beliefs. Mike was facing deep personal problems and severe character flaws as well as a history of people in his community condemning him. Not only did the belief that he was condemned represent the condemnation from his community but his own deeply complex and severe character flaws. In the case of John, on the other hand, the focus on Christ and Christ Consciousness represented a process by which the young man was able to meld his identity as a Christian with his identity as a hip bohemian artist.

Community dynamics can also play a part in the experiences of people in psychosis and post-psychosis, especially when the person is in a vulnerable condition. In the example of Will, after leaving Christianity Will was in post-psychosis and had tornado damage to his property. A fundamentalist disaster tourist said the tornado was act of god against sinners, causing Will to experience severe anxiety and have to use anti-anxiety pills. It is important to pay attention to the specifics of this situation. Not only is the disaster tourist using religion to condemn suffering people but Will has left Christianity after being raised in it and thereby has had condemning voices and emotions instilled in him, making him vulnerable to such condemnation. The anxiety response is not only a response to external events but also echoes past condemnations. The events are part of Will's struggle to practice his spirituality in line with his inner self and personal experience.

The face-to-face community, along with the family, instills emotions and voices into the person that, in combination with person's unique qualities, create mixtures of feelings and thoughts. This is the cluster of deeply held emotions that make up the personalities of young adults as they begin their lives. Each individual's psyche is made up of unique combinations of feelings and life events that play into the content of beliefs during psychosis. While in psychosis, the different emotions and voices take on lives of their own, seeming to be independent and greater than the person, often overwhelming the core person. Which feelings and voices are dominant at any time depend on where the person is on her or her journey through life and psychosis.

As evident from these examples, toxic family members, toxic community members and toxic aspects of larger world must be avoided and protected against to maintain safe place for sensitive people to flourish. In communities that are marked by centuries-long legacies of ethnic, religious, family and labor violence and oppression, as in the history of the United States, paying attention to the history of people and our families in the context of our community is central to the person's life journey he or she is on during the advent of psychosis.

Past traumas and shadow elements

In addition to aspects of one's personal world, past events, traumas and elements hidden in one's shadow can project themselves into the perceptions of someone in psychosis. In one case, an older person who had been stable for decades underwent a failed transition to a new medication, resulting in a brief period of psychosis. During this time the person developed the belief that people at her church were angry and judging her harshly because of her problems with mental illness, even though her friends were actively praying for her recovery. This passing delusion apparently had its origin in a trauma from her childhood when a nun had publically condemned her for a minor infraction and warned her harshly to "not be like" her father, who had suffered a mental collapse.

In a more complex example, during his early psychosis Mike recognized the significance of traumas from his past and negative family patterns that were being perpetuated in problems his adult life and marriage. Repeating family patterns is a common event in people's lives, especially in young people. During Mike's psychosis these problems were projected into his consciousness in highly symbolic and universal ways, as well as real life aspects of his situation. As Mike's psychosis and personality evolved he envisioned a resolution to the problems in the form of metaphorical beliefs and a magical quest. These confused insights became the basis for his personal transformation in post-psychosis.

Cultural scripts, icons and mythic stories

During psychosis, the highly fluid perception of reality within our hallucinations and delusions cause us to give up our normal, secular view of things. The phenomenological reasons for this are discussed in Chapter One of *Schizophrenia: A Blueprint for Recovery*. The consensus view of life as a secular, mundane process of physical events seems false and we turn to magical, iconic and mythic stories and scripts as fallback worldviews. These mystical and magical stories are much more capable of explaining events during psychosis and often become central to psychotic thinking.

The stories that people turn to can include other myths, such as when encounters with seemingly magical individuals are explained as being encounters with gods in disguise, a common event in Greek mythology. It is also common for mainstream stories, such as the Rapture, stories about Jesus, the Anti-Christ, and so forth, to take hold in the person's mind as an explanation for events. In the case of John, Mike and Theresa, religious stories played significant parts. John believed that he might be Jesus returning to Earth; Mike believed the Rapture was occurring and Theresa saw herself as being able to save the world through giving birth to a child, mimicking the story of the messiah.

These beliefs are part of the person's spiritual journey; seeing how personal meaning and real life events are connected to fantastic beliefs is essential in recognizing their meaning. These iconic, magical stories are ways we can express our experiences within the metaphorical and hallucinatory experiences of psychosis. Allowing people to discuss these stories and how they relate to our personal lives is central to recognizing their meaning and calming and communicating with people in psychosis.

World conditions and crises

The crises facing our industrialized civilization are a major part of the collective shadow of our time. While the concern by many people in psychosis about the end of the world may be linked to concerns that our personal world may fall apart, it is an unfortunate reality that there are many legitimate reasons to believe that within the next 50 years our civilization will face devastating crises. Currently our world civilization is facing the crisis of what anthropologist Marvin Harris called "the industrial bubble"—the rapid overconsumption of resources by our generation. Extensively well-researched and pertinent work, such as that by Lester Brown, various resource depletion experts and others indicate that our world civilization is racing towards resource depletion and pollution toxicity. Meanwhile, by all meaningful measures, the United States appears to be in the grip of the infamous cultural decay of collapsing civilizations, ranging from widespread use of porn to wanton abuse of power-over-others to diminishing resources devoted to families and children to a hedonistic apathy by many ordinary people that distract them from facing our collective crises.

Mentally ill people are oftentimes much more concerned about larger world problems than the ordinary person. I personally see this as showing how mentally ill people can have qualities that are superior to mainstream people, even though and possibly because we are mentally ill. The concern shown by mentally ill people about our collective fate is much greater than that of the mainstream people I have worked with for 25 years. To me, this shows a spiritual desire to help humanity that many in the mainstream sorely lack. Sadly, our illnesses prevent us from realizing our ideals of making the world a better place.

Given the very real challenges facing our civilization, concerns about the larger world expressed by mentally ill people should be recognized as potentially legitimate. It is not uncommon for mentally ill people to seek impractical or magical solutions to these real world problems. Acknowledging the reality of the situation and the good intentions of the mentally ill person can be central in respecting them as well-meaning and sincere people.

Also being aware of how personal issues can be expressed with macro-level icons can help outsiders understand an individual's personal life and the beliefs she or he express. For example, one white man in psychosis was married to a black woman and developed the belief that the Deity was Jah, the African god of Rastafarians. In doing so, the man was seeking to make sacred the struggles and challenges of his wife in a national and international European-dominated society with centuries of racist oppression.

SOME COMMON FEATURES OF PSYCHOSIS

The purpose of this section is to show real life reasons people cling to delusions and legitimate experiences of people in psychosis. It is an extension of Chapter One of *Schizophrenia: A Blueprint for Recovery*, which describes the building of psychosis as the result of ongoing hallucinations. In the section below, four elements commonly experienced by people in psychosis—synchronicity, accurate intuitions, symbolic beliefs and meaningful coincidences—are reviewed to give the reader a sense for the inner experiences, thoughts and feelings of a person in psychosis. In many cases, these events have real aspects in the world around us. However, people in psychosis often misinterpret them as having far greater significance to far more people than they actually do.

Synchronicity

In Western psychological thought synchronicity, the coincidence between thoughts and events was first identified by Jung. Prophetic dreams are a commonly recognized example of synchronicity. Accounts of synchronicity are prominent in ancient Western history. Just before his assassination on the Ides of March, Caesar's wife had a dream warning of his death during that time and is quoted as telling Caesar, "Beware the Ides of March."

In an example from Greek history, when the city-state of Athens was threatened by an overwhelming force from the Persian Empire in 480 BC, Athenians sent envoys to the Oracle at Delphi for a prophecy. The Oracle at Delphi stated that "All will fail save the wooden wall," which the Athenian leader Themistocles interpreted as indicating the

Athenian naval fleet, made of ships of wood, would be key to success. The Oracle also grimly advised, "O holy Salamis, you will be the death of many a woman's son..." A trap was set for the Persian navy at Salamis and the Greek navy was victorious, devastating the Persian fleet and forcing the Persians into retreat.

In our contemporary culture, little if any value is publically placed on such stories, however, synchronicity is a common occurrence in daily life. It can be observed and studied without reliance on the outside world or on supposed experts.

During psychosis, it is common for people to become fascinated by synchronicities, seeing them as indicating a spiritual world and the possibility of mind over matter. To understand the mind set of people viewing these events, there are a series of examples below that come from my own life in post-psychosis. As these events are recounted, I will also note how a person in psychosis might interpret them.

In the first example, my family had just gone on vacation when we received a call that my stepson's dog, who had been left in the care of friends, had escaped and been lost. A friend of my stepson, back in our hometown, heard that the dog was lost and that night dreamed that he would find the dog. The next day, he walked down the street and asked people if they had seen the dog. The second person he spoke to said that a friend of his had found the dog and was keeping her in his backyard for safety. Our friend's dream had come true and he had found my stepson's dog.

I was talking to my stepson's friend about his dream a couple of years later and he indicated that he had prophetic dreams fairly often. He said that he had been working to fix a radio of his for a year and a few nights before he dreamed that he finally was able to fix the radio. He got up the next day and was able to fix the radio.

Interestingly, my stepson's friend had a roommate who has schizophrenia. Though stable during that time, had the young man with schizophrenia told his psychiatrist about his roommate's prophetic dreams, he might have been thought to be delusional.

A normal person who is willing to believe in prophetic dreams would take these events as proof that dreams can be prophetic. A person in psychosis, however, would likely to jump to conclusions about the significance of the dreams. He or she could easily believe that the dreams had come true because all dreams come true, so everything that she or he dreamed of would manifest at some point.

In another example of a series of synchronicities, one Thursday during the spring my wife wondered aloud if a friend of ours from the West Coast, who visited regularly during the spring and summer, was going to come soon. The next day, unknown to us, my stepson was in his home when his dog began barking wildly, which she did only when the friend from the West Coast was around. My stepson thought to himself that his dog was barking as if the friend was there. Two days later, I looked out a window and I saw our friend from the West Coast walking up to our house. We later told my stepson about my wife's thinking of the friend just before he arrived and my stepson told us about his dog barking wildly.

To someone who is mystically oriented, these events would indicate that intuition is a fairly common phenomenon, including in animals. To a person in psychosis, however, beliefs that are more elaborate might occur, including that the energy of the friend from the West Coast had preceded him or that the friend had been thinking of visiting and his thoughts had triggered the events.

In another, much more serious example, I had a synchronicity about the health of a coworker. The coworker, who worked in a different building but for the same customer as I did, was dealing with a heavy workload. One Monday I wondered how she was handling the pressure and I heard myself think, "I think the coworker will die." It is common for random thoughts to enter my mind, so I did not think much of the matter.

Unknown to me the coworker was sick at home with a ruptured appendix. She did not realize her appendix had ruptured and was waiting for her family to return from vacation to seek medical help. On Tuesday night, my coworker's boss and a fellow worker went to her home and insisted she go to the emergency room. On Wednesday morning our work group received an email explaining that the coworker had emergency laparoscopic surgery the night before to remove her appendix. Suddenly aware of the true nature of the situation and remembering my thought, I began to earnestly pray for her health and well-being. Meanwhile, a second coworker read the email and immediately thought to herself that our severely ill coworker might die. Like me, she began to pray for our coworker's health.

On Friday, we received another email saying the coworker had been life-flighted to the Ohio State University

Medical Center because she had pieces of her appendix left inside of her. She underwent another laparoscopic surgery and then a full surgery to fully remove the toxic tissue. Though she survived, she spent weeks away from work and required months to reach a point near full recovery. The week after the surgeries, my coworkers and I were discussing the situation and the other coworker who had thought that the gravely ill coworker might die and I discovered we had the same thought and were both praying very hard since that time.

A mystical person would probably think that these events indicate a "universal mind" or general spirit that connects people and allows intuition to occur. A person in psychosis, however, might take the predictions literally and believe that the coworker had really died and had been reborn or replaced by a doppelganger or clone of some sort.

It is important to note the all events above occurred in groups of people, so if a person who is in psychosis witnessed them there would be people who could confirm all of these events. If the person in psychosis told someone in the mental health system about these events, it is likely that he or she would be thought to be delusional. However, if pressed to disbelieve her or his real life experiences, the person in psychosis would be driven away from the treatment team and feel confident that they and the other eyewitnesses are perceiving events correctly and it is the treatment team who are mistaken about reality. And, in these examples, that would be true.

In the next two examples, I will review the synchronicities from point of view of how person in psychosis might behave in response to witnessing them. In the hallucinatory perception of psychosis, reality appears much more fluid and changeable than it appears in ordinary perception, so we often come to believe that there are various forms of mind over matter that we can use to communicate, share energy with others and even permanently change reality. Synchronicities seem to be indicators of ways to shape reality through thoughts, words and small actions.

In the first case, I was playing a CD of a local Old Time String band and while it played I went downstairs to our kitchen. While I was in the kitchen I missed hearing a song on the CD called "Darlin' Cory." I like the song and after the CD finished I replayed the CD, pressing the track number to start at "Darlin' Cory." The next day I was in our kitchen and my mother-in-law had a local radio station on in her bedroom next to our kitchen. The DJ announced that he was about to play a song by a local Old Time String band and then played "Darlin' Cory." That was the first time in my life I have ever heard "Darlin' Cory" on the radio and it was more than five years later before I heard the song on the radio again.

If a person in psychosis witnessed this synchronicity, it is likely that she or he would believe that the act of replaying "Darling Cory" had resulted in it being played on radio. The person would probably think that magical energy had emanated from replaying the song and this energy had entered the mind of the DJ and caused him to play the song. The person in psychosis would probably also believe that magical energy emanated from the radio station broadcasting this song and this energy had been shared with people throughout the area.

Because of the believed sharing of energy through the song, the person would see replaying songs as a way to transmit the energy and message of songs, both in mundane and magical ways. After this the person might begin to replay a song that he or she felt was particularly important, seeking to repeat the synchronicity and spread the energy to others.

In another example of synchronicity, I happened to have a brief discussion with a bank teller about the importance of genetic diversity in dog breeding to prevent birth defects. This led us to discuss how the drive for racial purity in humans by racists actually results in genetic defects because defects tend to occur in populations with limited diversity in DNA. I left the bank and within a minute I saw an interracial couple walking down the street holding hands.

A person in psychosis would probably believe that the conversation with the teller had brought interracial couple into her or his life. The couple might be from another reality, might have been created spontaneously by the conversation or might have been somehow drawn closer to person through the conversation. If person were for integration, he or she would repeat the conversation several times to generate more interracial couples. If the person were against integration, he or she would try to stop conversations like these.

For people who are deep in psychosis and have developed complex delusional frameworks, we will believe from synchronicities that thinking, feeling or doing the wrong thing in a seemingly mundane situation can result in accidently bringing about a terrible catastrophe. In my own case, while in a mental hospital in the fall of 1985, I had a brief encounter with another mentally ill person that confused me. I was not sure what the woman wanted from me, she seemed distressed and I felt that whatever I tried to do was wrong. The next morning the television broadcasted news of a horrendously destructive earthquake that had devastated Mexico City. I felt that my bumbling with the woman in need had caused the earthquake to occur. When I discussed this with another person in post-psychosis years later the other fellow indicated that he had a similar delusion about the Oklahoma City bombing that occurred while he was in psychosis in the mid-1990s.

Accurate intuitions

Accurate intuitions, like prophetic dreams, are synchronicities which give us information from out of the blue, often in the form of feelings or unusual events that bring sudden thoughts to mind. The accurate intuitions discussed in this section mainly occurred during psychosis and are drawn primarily from post-psychotic surveys I conducted. Psychosis, which is similar to a dream-like state, seems to increase the likelihood that people have accurate intuitions. Because of these accurate intuitions, along with other insights, the experience of psychosis is taken to be a heightened awareness and all of our unusual experiences are taken as meaningful and important.

In one case from the post-psychotic surveys, a woman reported that she was riding a horse when she saw a horseman in long robes. She felt she was being told to return home and stable her horse, which she did. Shortly afterwards a violent storm blew up. Had she been riding during the storm her horse might have panicked and thrown her, potentially resulting in serious injury or even her own death. The woman appreciated the importance and value of the message she had received and only after she returned from psychosis did she realize that the man in long robes had been a hallucination. The hallucinatory event may have saved her life.

In a second example from the post-psychotic surveys, Will reported his "precognition" frequently gave him accurate intuitions. During his treatment, he predicted that his therapist's wife would have a car accident. She, in fact, did have a car accident. Instead of recognizing the accuracy of the intuition and the good will behind the warning, the therapist called the police and had them investigate Will for possibly trying to harm his wife. It is noteworthy that not only did the therapist lack insight about his client's accurate intuition but he also had unwarranted fear of the man he was supposed to help.

In a third example from the post-psychotic surveys, Haley was in deep psychosis in a mental hospital was talking on the phone with a friend who she had not seen in months. The friend was overweight and had been trying to diet despite a fondness for chocolate. Haley smelled chocolate, even though none was around, and she asked her old friend if she had been eating chocolate. Her friend admitted that she had been eating chocolate and had not been able to lose weight.

As a follow-up to this, I spoke to Haley, now in post-psychosis, about this and she related that she had been talking on the phone with her father and had, once again, smelled chocolate. Haley asked her father if he was eating chocolate and he, in fact, was. It is significant that this reoccurring event, fitting the definition of an olfactory hallucination, has been a reliable indicator what friend and family were eating.

During my own psychosis, I was having a conversation with a dorm mate in an enclosed room. Unknown to the man, I was attempting to unlock spiritual energy within him through ritual use of words with hidden meanings. I finished my conversation with him and left the room, but as I walked down the hall I thought of one more thing to say to unlock the energy.

I turned around but before I could step back towards the door I heard his voice through the door say, "Let me open the door." The wall between us was made of concrete blocks and the door was solid and neither the wall nor the door had windows or openings, so there was no way I could hear or see the fellow. I paused, thinking that his soul was saying that he wanted to "open the door" to the spiritual energy I was seeking to unlock within him. Moments later he walked through the door into the hallway where I was waiting. I finished my conversation with him, convinced that I had heard what he was thinking at a deep level.

After this incident I began to hear people's voices coming from beside their heads. Neither their mouth nor jaws were moving, but the voices sounded like their speaking voices and what was said seemed to fit their personality. Given the accurate intuition, I believed I was beginning to hear people's thoughts. I did not believe I could read minds, however, because I was skeptical and thought if I could read people's minds I would be able to hear all their thoughts at will. Accordingly, I believed that if I undertook spiritual practices to unlock my own spiritual energy I would someday be able to read minds.

In a final example, I happened to be at a conference when I met a young man who was in post-psychosis. He and I had brief conversations and at the beginning of the second or third of these conversations he surprised me with three very accurate intuitions about me and my life at that time. I was struck by his remarkable intuitive ability and also by his incredibly gentle and sensitive nature.

During my presentation at the conference, to help illustrate the experiences of people in psychosis, I described this young man's remarkable abilities and suggested that we consider what he might experience walking down a city street, where he might see people who are addicted to drugs, people without homes, people who victims of abuse and people who are abusive, as well as many others struggling with the normal trials and tribulations of life. With his sensitivity, the simple act of walking down the street could be extremely powerful and potentially very difficult. Imagining his experiences as someone who would have his accurate intuitions projected in symbolic form into his hallucinations and delusions can give one a sense of the nature of psychosis for sensitive people like this remarkable young man. Given his abilities and experiences, it is completely understandable that in post-psychosis he has had to learn how to deal with feelings of anxiety that affect him every so often.

Symbolic beliefs

Many seemingly delusional beliefs are symbolic references to our personal world that we misinterpret as applying to all people throughout eternity. This is often related to our hallucinatory perceptions that the world is much more magical and fluid than we previously thought. We often pick up cultural symbols and have experiences in which we make personal contact with cultural icons, ranging from religious entities like angels or demons to celebrities to aliens and other extraordinary beings. With this backdrop and within the dream-like experience of psychosis, we relate to the world as if symbolic observations are literal and universal truths.

In one example, a conservative Christian woman with bipolar mania causing psychosis became concerned that her children's GI Joe war toys were satanic. She saw the enemy organization of GI Joe, COBRA, as referring to the serpent in the Garden of Eden and the stars as pentacles used by Satanists. She took away the GI Joe toys that had these images or references, thinking that she was protecting her children from Satan.

The woman was experiencing a magical interpretation of collective cultural symbols. The choice by the GI Joe Company to have "COBRA" as the enemy was certainly thoroughly discussed by the marketing team and was probably consciously based on traditional negative associations with snakes in Western culture. The relationship of snakes to the ultimate Christian evil was not accidental; rather it was almost certainly a marketing ploy using cultural associations to evoke feelings of evil.

Why the woman associated stars with pentacles rather than with the US flag can have different answers depending on the woman's life situation. Possibilities include that the association is simply a generalization from COBRA; a result of the woman's focus as conservative Christianity; caused by negative feelings about the US government and/or culture due to issues like abortion or based on negative experiences with people in authority, especially those associated with stars, such as people in the military or the police.

In long-term psychosis it is likely that these beliefs would become more general. The stars as pentacles could easily lead to the belief that the stars (pentacles) on the US flag means that the government was founded or taken over by Satanists. It is important to recognize that the woman's beliefs arose from her becoming conscious of unconscious cultural symbols and ascribing magical and spiritual causes to these connections. Cultural symbols and their use in marketing and communication is common way many people are manipulated. When people in psychosis recognize these real symbols we often leap to delusional conclusions because these iconic symbols are being used to affect people around us.

In another example, a person in psychosis believed that government was watching him. The person lived in a wooded rural area and when helicopters would fly overhead, he thought they were government agents spying on him. He would run into the woods to avoid the agents seeing him.

While this belief appears to be a typical paranoid delusion, the belief actually reflected the context of the person's life in exaggerated terms. At that time, most of the helicopters in this person's area were police who were searching for pot fields hidden in the woods. The person smoked pot during this time, so it is a simple leap to the false conclusion that the police in the helicopters were spying on him rather than just looking for pot fields.

In addition, the father of the person in psychosis was a leftist scholar during the Cold War and volunteered with peace and justice groups that were commonly seen as subversive by the US government. Given the hostility of the US government towards dissenters and the long record of spying on those who objected to the handling of the Cold War, it is almost certain that the father has an FBI file and may have been watched at times. Again, the leap to the conclusion that the helicopters contained government agents spying on the person in psychosis is not very far. With the grandiose nature of psychotic thinking and the generalization of personal facts into exaggerated beliefs, the connection between the personal reality and the delusion is obvious.

Other examples of experiences that are symbolic or coming from the context of the person's life are found in the post-psychotic surveys of Haley and Will. Both individuals describe how events and reading material in real life were mimicked by hallucinatory or delusional events in their psychosis. Haley reported that Biblical passages she read were often seemingly mimicked in events around her within a few hours or days of the reading. Will reported that when he heard his religious group speaking in tongues the words and voices would often re-appear in his hallucinations shortly afterwards.

It appears that psychosis contains a process of echoing events, projecting real life stimuli into hallucinations and delusions. This echoing, combined with exaggeration and symbolization of one's life into psychotic content, creates an ongoing appearance of reality supporting the delusions we experience. We feel our delusional beliefs are true because of their close relationship to our reality and also allows us to gain insight into our lives through beliefs that both represent and exaggerate our personal world. Misinterpreting these metaphorical references to our lives as universal and literal events creates a layer of confusion that overlays our potential insights.

Coincidence and meaning

The role of meaningful coincidences in psychosis is prominent in the retelling of these events by those in postpsychosis. In the case of Mike in the second passage, he tells of "receiving messages from strange events and coincidences" that gave him a grim and accurate prediction for the future. In another case, a person told a story of being separated from a friend at a huge amphitheater during a rock concert and being taken by an urge to walk down a long aisle. This urge led him directly to his friend and gave the person in psychosis a sense that there was something mystical going on.

John, in the second passage, tells the story of coincidences that surrounded him picking up a hitchhiking itinerant musician named Leaf. Leaf had the words "Live Free" tattooed on his fingers and John and Leaf discussed the philosophy that Leaf was embodying in his life. This made an impression on John who, at the time, was a young man seeking to expand himself as a person and artist.

Though not being from the area, Leaf had made an impression on a friend of John as well. The next day John's friend brought up Leaf, a musician she had met while visiting a city of the same name as theirs in a different state. John was surprised and he and his friend discovered that they had met the same person by chance. Shortly thereafter John went through a psychotic crisis with terrifying delusions during his arrest and ride to hospital. In this moment of dread, John remembered the coincidences surrounding Leaf and saw them as signs of the importance of Leaf's philosophy and of mysticism, giving him strength amidst the crisis.

After release from hospital, John want for a long walk and saw "Leaf" sprayed on door, giving him an even greater sense for the importance of the events and of mysticism in his life. All of the events were confirmed by non-psychotic individuals, giving John concrete reasons to feel that these events were indeed significant to him.

In my own case, I noticed coincidences and synchronicity during my psychosis and made a choice to follow coincidences based on names. During that time I was living in a town called Athens that, despite its name, had only one family from Greece in it. The family owned a restaurant with apartments over it and since my own last name was "Greek" and I was living in Athens I decided to center myself in the energy of my life in the community by taking an apartment over the Greek restaurant. I felt I was fulfilling some sort of destiny.

When I moved in I met two neighbors who, despite knowing I was psychotic, accepted me. I did not realize at the time that I was hallucinating and delusional, but they did. Rather than keeping away from me they decided to try to provide me aid. Beyond keeping me company and being friends, they tried to protect me from social predators, ease my anxieties and, at one point, gave me a guided meditation that was effective in relaxing me and giving me a sense of strength.

During this time I was in a store with my two neighbors and I had a hallucination in which the world swirled around us. Only the three of us remained steady and clear. From this I believed we were the same soul during some incarnation and we were still deeply connected.

Shortly after this I fell into crisis and was taken from my apartment by Mom. After a period of searching, my parents decided I should go to a mental hospital, which I voluntarily entered.

After about three years, I was stable and returned to Athens to finish my college degrees. Despite neither of my old friends being from the town or going to college, I happened to meet one of them walking down the street. They were still roommates in another apartment house.

During this time we once again became daily companions. By chance they moved into a house with a backyard adjacent to my backyard and during the year they and I visited each other constantly. This was the first new non-mentally ill circle of friends I had after I accepted my diagnosis.

It is noteworthy that these friends were bookends to my intensive mental health treatment; they were daily companions immediately prior to my hospitalizations and were daily companions at the beginning of my return to mainstream society. They were kind and helpful to me throughout our friendship and we felt a genuine affection for each other. There is no doubt that their presence in my life was very helpful. Had I not chosen to pursue coincidences I would have never met them.

PSYCHOSIS AS AN UNRECOGNIZED VISION QUEST

Vision quests, shamanism and remarkable events in altered states

In non-Western cultures, vision quests are intentional means to create "visions" of unseen and future worlds. By Western definitions, a vision quest is a state where physical exhaustion is used to generate hallucinations that are then analyzed for meaning. While most Westerners do not believe that vision quests are useful or meaningful, there is evidence that altered states can produce surprisingly remarkable and useful events.

In US history, probably the most significant vision quest was the vision of the Lakota victory at Little Big Horn by Lakota medicine man Sitting Bull. Documented at a sacred site by the Lakota people which has since been made a national historical site,[1] the vision quest occurred during the Lakota Sun Dance ceremony about two weeks before the defeat of Custer in 1876. Descriptions indicate that Sitting Bull lacerated his arms extensively and danced continuously for hours to bring on the vision, which he described as seeing dead enemy warriors falling from the sky. Seeing

---

[1] see http://www.nps.gov/nhl/IMR/Montana_HPP_2012.pdf

this vision informed him and the Lakota people of the impending victory against the European invaders.[2]

Another example of remarkable abilities attributed to Native American medicine men comes from an account in Never Cry Wolf, Farley Mowat's story of his study of wolves in the far north of Canada. While in an isolated region of the countryside, the Inuit shaman Ootek told Mowat that the wolves were calling to each other that humans were coming to visit Mowat, including Europeans. A couple of days later Mowat was surprised by unexpected visitors to his remote camp. Ootek explained to Mowat that as a young child he had been identified as someone who would become a medicine man and he was placed in a wolf den for several days. Since that time Ootek had come to understand the messages that the wolves sent each other through their howling. By hearing the wolves' calls Ootek had learned the visitors were coming.

While these stories sound unbelievable to many secular Westerners, there is evidence from our modern culture that altered states can bring about positive results. During his career as a major league pitcher, Dock Ellis pitched one no-hitter. Years later, Ellis went public with the story that he had taken LSD prior to his historic no-hitter. Despite experiencing hallucinations and odd occurrences during the game, Ellis's skill appears to have been aided by his altered state, allowing him to achieve, if only that one time, what few major league pitchers have ever achieved.

---

[2] Utley, Robert M. *Sitting Bull: The Life and Times of an American Patriot* (pp. 137-139); *The Lance and the Shield: The Life and Times of Sitting Bull.* (pp. 122-124).

In addition to these indications that altered states can aid ability, insights in trance states is very common in spiritual traditions. Spontaneous speech attributed to other entities is claimed to have generated lucid and popular literature for centuries, ranging from the poetic verses of the 7th century Qur'an to numerous New Age books, including the very popular Orin and DaBen series. In looking at the Orin and DaBen series, books such as Spiritual Growth contain a high level of psychological insight that many people with advanced degrees in psychology and other fields would find intriguing and useful.

From the Western, secular viewpoint, these references indicate little of value; however this viewpoint is a small minority view compared to other cultures. Non-western views of spirituality and mysticism are very different from modern Western secularism. In particular, in many cultures there is often no division between religion and science or between religion and mysticism.

While Western thought has been greatly affected by conflict between religion and secular views, I suggest that deistic and atheistic Western counseling assumptions are at odds with internal experience of psychosis and vision quest. This is not to say that those in psychosis are experiencing a vision quest or necessarily have enhanced abilities; rather, psychosis can be thought of as an unintended and unrecognized vision quest.

Some people who experience psychosis as vision quest prone

In looking for evidence that exhaustion can generate hallucinations, the experiences of soldiers who undergo

Army Ranger (Officer) training are significant. Army Ranger training is made up of weeks intensive physical trials in which trainees are parachuted into swamps in Florida and forced marched out in battle-like conditions, followed by miles of running in the summer Georgia sun in full gear, following by being airlifted into the Western Rockies and parachuted onto remote mountains where they are again force marched in battle-like conditions. This training is an ongoing test of physical and mental endurance.

In speaking with those who have undergone this arduous training, soldiers report that hallucinations are common. In one case, a veteran with bipolar disorder retold how he was ordered by an officer to set up a machine gun nest at the edge of a cliff. He grabbed his gun and ran full speed towards the cliff, only to be tackled by a fellow soldier who convinced him the officer was a hallucination. In a second case, a non-mentally ill vet ran five miles in Georgia heat, completing the run while others dropped out, but then experienced hallucinations and thought he was surrounded by enemies. In what could have been a very dangerous situation, a buddy he trusted was able to calm him and help him realize that he was hallucinating.

Both soldiers reported that "everyone" who went through Ranger training experienced hallucinations at some point. The second person indicated that he watched his fellow trainees and foresaw whether they would hallucinate earlier or later during the training based on his sense of the different susceptibility of the fellow trainees to having hallucinations.

Many who experience psychosis may be "vision quest prone." In other words, we experience hallucinations with less physical, emotional and cognitive stress than other individuals. For example, in the story of Theresa in the second passage, her second experience of psychosis appears to have begun during a physically and emotionally arduous weeklong course that included heavy exercise and lack of sleep. In similar ways, traumas, social and emotional stresses, physical illnesses and intensive mental work may lead vision quest prone people to experience psychosis when others would not.

Hypothetical relationship between vision quests and psychosis

In the hallucinatory state of psychosis, personal, family, community and collective shadows and our personal struggles are projected into a delusional framework. Once we are deeply experiencing psychosis, we do not recognize our altered state, resulting in misperception of personal symbolic hallucinatory events as literal physical events with universal meaning. Looking at the common events of psychosis described previously, including synchronicity, accurate intuitions, symbolic beliefs and meaningful coincidences, we can see that we are led to believe in a mystical spirituality as an empirically valid result of our personal journey.

In looking at narratives of psychosis, we see psychosis often leads to learning and integrating our life lessons. This is illustrated in the cases of John, Mike and Theresa in the second passage. In even more important forms of personal growth, the cases of Mike and Theresa allowed them to be able to share their lives with a life-long soul mate. In these stories there is substantial evidence that psychosis can greatly benefit a person who undergoes it.

There are very important differences between vision quests and psychoses which are crucial to understanding why vision quests can be normal parts of life for some while psychosis can be extremely debilitating events for others.

The key differences are:

- Psychosis does not have clear boundaries in time, so we who experience it do not realize when it is beginning or ending.
- Hallucinations are not recognized as non-consensus events in psychosis, causing them to be taken for literal events with universal and eternal implications.
- Psychosis occurs over long periods of time, causing ongoing misinterpretation of events to be very substantial and grow into a very complex delusional framework.
- The delusional framework tends to be more often symbolic expressions of personal, rather than universal or tribal, concerns, making the perspective much narrower.
- Psychosis in Western society occurs in a culture without an understanding of the validity and boundaries of vision quests, resulting in a lack of cultural knowledge about helpful responses to these events.

Because of these crucial differences between vision quests and psychosis, those who experience an unrecognized and unintended vision quest often need help in determining what is and is not reality. At the same time, because of the tremendously complex cultural knowledge surrounding vision quests in the cultures that practice them, Westerners like me do not have the ability understand shamanism simply because we have experienced psychosis.

Additional theoretical construct from spirituality

In depth psychology theory such as created by Freud and Jung, there is a view of more and less conscious and unconscious selves in the parallel concepts of the Persona/Superego and Shadow/Id. In both of these views of human being, there are some ideas that people have an inner drive for some positive self-attainment, but this discussion is limited. In this passage, this viewpoint has allowed discussion of disharmonies within and around the person as creating a desire to transcend personal limitations.

However, Western secular psychological thought is notably pessimistic about the nature of the person. A case in point comes from a workshop on jobs and recovery that I attended at a conference a few years ago. During the workshop the presenter used Maslow's hierarchy of needs to describe the desires that lead people to work, with self-actualization as the highest attainment.

Though Maslow's work is seen one of the most optimistic views of humanity in Western psychology, the discussion during the workshop showed that it was inadequate in explaining why people wanted to work. A fellow attendee and I both indicated that one of the reasons we worked was "because we love others in our lives."

"You work so you can feel loved by others," the presenter replied, following Maslow's explanation of our needs.

No, we explained, we worked because the money we made allowed us to feed, clothe, and provide shelter and happiness to those we loved. By making those we loved happy and healthy by our work, we were happy because our work made things possible for those we dearly loved. We would rather work and provide those we love with what they need in this hard world than have them suffer because we aren't working. Maslow's idealistic view of humanity was still far too self-involved and isolated from people loving our families and friends to understand the altruism that is central to many people's family and community lives.

In place of this selfish and isolated view of people, spiritual thinking discusses what is variously called the Oversoul, the Deep or Deeper Self, the Higher Self, and the Deity-within or the Atman. This is in essence our most spiritually powerful aspect, our soul or spiritual connection to the sacred part of the universe. The Deity-within intervenes occasionally in our life to make big decisions, though at the time these decisions often seem to be brought on by chance events. This aspect of our spirit is primarily concerned with spiritual rather than material well-being, which can make it very impractical. However, the concern of this spirituality is not simply a relationship between the person and the Deity, but our effect on the web of life around us.

It is important to understand that this spiritual part of us has the desire to bring about a highly spiritual "heaven on Earth" in the web of life around us. This drive is an oftentimes unrecognized and suppressed aspect of people's innate being, beaten down by hardships and day-to-day trials and toil of modern life. Even so, this inner drive for a better life for ourselves and the people we love and even the world as a whole can be seen in people and their lives, including in secular-minded people who work to help others.

From a spiritual viewpoint, most people are born into double binds that we are supposed to overcome through psychological and spiritual growth. This process is our life lesson and is part of the spiritual purpose of our lives. Learning and applying our life lesson is central to living a spiritual life. For many post-psychotic people, psychosis was a time during which we learned our life lesson and received the emotional drive to transform our lives.

In cases where psychosis is not the result of torture or other similar severe trauma, psychosis can often occur as a choice by the "deep self" or soul of the person with the intention of sparking a spiritual quest to bring about a transformation in the person and surrounding web of life. This choice, a gamble in which the life of the person and those around him or her are placed in jeopardy, is an attempt for the deep self to dramatically alter the person's life course for the better. In the state of psychosis, this highly idealistic, impractical drive manifests as a symbolic quest that is simultaneously delusional and symbolically meaningful to the spiritual goals of the deep self. This perspective must seem bizarre and nonsensical to many reading this, but it is brought up because for many who have experienced psychosis the events cannot be understood without recognizing this crucial spiritual viewpoint. This viewpoint is similar to those of many peers in peer movement, especially in the works of Paris Williams.

In this perspective, the "purpose" of psychosis is to bring unconscious elements to consciousness so this knowledge can be used to help transform the person's life. In some cases this choice is due to the unconscious controlling and destroying one's personal life, both spirituality and materially, as appears to be the situation with Mike. In other cases, such as John and Will, the purpose appears to be to bring heightened awareness of abilities and spirituality. And, as indicated before, psychosis can also lead to life-long partners and families, as with Mike and Theresa. This last attainment can be argued to be one of the highest attainments of a person's spiritual goals in this life.

This radical view of psychosis may not always apply nor be a sign of an inferior person or a horrible trauma to overcome. In some cases, psychoses may be caused by purely physiological events, such as drug use, a genetic predisposition or substantial physical or emotional stress. In other cases, as in the journey of John, the amount of trauma and negative life conditions prior to psychosis do not fit into a remedial model where a person's suffering soul yearns to overcome horrible conditions; rather these instances suggest that psychosis can be part of a deep soul yearning to have a life that is more meaningful and dynamically aware than the average person's life. As such, it most clearly has parallels to voluntary vision quests of self-discovery and spiritual attainments.

For those who do not wish to be "burdened" by seemingly unempirical spiritual ideas, the view of psychosis as instigating deep changes in the person can be seen as simply recognizing the nature of the experience. The projection of our life content into psychosis causes the most important aspects of our lives to be dramatically highlighted. Parts of our lives that cause deep pain—ranging from personal trauma or failings to real, large world crises—are thrown into our consciousness and made unbearable by the intensity and clarity of the challenge. The psychotic experience becomes a catalyst for transformation. Regardless of how the psychosis is viewed, this catalyst can potentially manifest a much better life for the person and those around him or her. This process of self-discovery and fulfillment is illustrated in the five stories in the second passage.

Spiritual Journeys

The following material is drawn in large part from post-psychotic surveys that were first discussed in Appendix C of *Schizophrenia: A Blueprint for Recovery*. About half of the post-psychotic survey respondents reported nightmarish experiences while the other half reported transcendent experiences and spoke highly of the experience. Those with nightmarish experiences, such as Haley in this section, described psychosis as "a number one enemy" (G-4) and something that caused them to imagine demons (G-9). Others indicated that psychosis was "a gift as well as a blessing" (John) an experience that gave them insight which psychiatric treatment interfered with (G-10). While the nightmarish scenarios conform to traditional expectations of the content of psychosis, the transcendent experiences point to possible interpretations of psychosis that have been overlooked in the past.

Nightmarish scenarios often contain some combination of trauma, severe character flaws, harshly judgmental religion and stress. These seem to build on each other, where trauma has created a character flaw that people keep hidden in their shadows and which people react to through having personas that make harsh judgments about themselves and others. At the same time, the character flaws create stressful situations and bring negative events and people with complementary character flaws into the person's life, creating problems that feed the negative qualities of the psychosis. This combination creating at first a nightmarish scenario that evolved into a positive experience is seen in the story of Mike.

It is important to not see the nightmarish scenarios as a "bad" version of the transcendent experiences nor the transcendent experiences as "delusional rationalizations" of post-psychotic people covering their dysfunction. For the purpose of understanding people's experiences during psychosis and aiding recovery and transformation, the accounts that people in post-psychosis give about their experiences should be taken as accurate and meaningful description of psychosis in their unique experience. It is essential to respect each story so that we can find the full breadth and depth of what people experience during what is called "psychosis."

Looking for the relationship between a person's beliefs and her or his life context makes it possible to help envision a healing resolution for the trauma, stresses and disharmonies that underlie the psychosis. Implementing a healing resolution in the person's real life will help reduce stress and psychotic symptoms, reduce paranoia, increase trust and cooperation and begin the journey of transformation.

For the purpose of this review, the stories being retold are mainly transcendent in nature. In these stories, psychosis can be recognized as a spiritual journey towards a healing resolution. The individuals telling the stories often describe finding meaning and moving towards personal development and spiritual growth through their embracing insights while eliminating confusion.

To help aid the accuracy of the stories that followed, the post-psychotic essays completed by Haley, Will and John were re-ordered in chronological order and comments and additional material was solicited. Each person added some additional material to the original essay. Mike's essay was written in 2013 for this work. For Theresa's material, which was taken directly from Paris's Williams' *Rethinking Madness* and chronologically ordered, was sent to Theresa who reviewed it for accuracy. These stories are told as much as possible in the words of the person who experienced them, including typos, misspelling and grammatical errors.

These spiritual journeys seem to have two main, readily observable aspects. Firstly, they tend to be movements from a disharmonious web of life into a more harmonious and personally meaningful web of life. Secondly, the person's spiritual beliefs, practices and affiliations prior to psychosis change to different beliefs, practices and affiliations in post-psychosis. These two general, large scale changes tend to be brought about by recognition of aspects their inner self and nature that had been previously unconscious or unacknowledged. In the cases detailed here, these changes are regarded by the people as ultimately beneficial to them. The spiritual journeys also contain some or all of the following. Psychosis expressing personal identity; psychosis allowing a person to have spiritual faith not available elsewhere; and psychosis providing insight to personal growth.

By studying these events, there is the possibility of refining therapeutic approaches to aid the spiritual growth of people in psychosis. By doing so, it may be possible to not only calm and stabilize a person through psychosis but also to create positive changes that makes the person happier, healthier, more well-adjusted and a more responsible member of her or his community than prior to psychosis. This transformation, instigated by psychosis, will hopefully one day be seen as important as and as a crucial partner to recovery for people experiencing psychosis.

HALEY

From addiction and nihilism to deliverance and renewal

In her post-psychotic survey, Haley describes her psychosis as powerfully affected by her miraculous religious conversion and her quest to save the souls of those around her. This journey begins in her personal world, where Haley's childhood was marked by severe trauma, isolation and dysfunction that initially lead her into drug addiction and beliefs in Satanism.

Personal world

As a young person, Haley was a daughter of a mother who suffered from bipolar syndrome, smoked cigarettes and was alcoholic, appears to have had a personality disorder with flares of temper and emotional abuse. The father was somewhat emotionally absent, warm and congenial but enabling the mother's addictions and doing little to counteract the emotional impact of his wife.

Haley writes,

> When I was a child I felt isolated and alone, I was withdrawn and shy. I felt that most kids

> in school were making fun of me, and I felt bad about myself most of the time. My father was a fun person that I would play and have fun with, but with no siblings, an alcoholic mother, and no family members nearby; I was sad and lonely.

In 8th grade, Haley began to be pressured and coerced into sexual activity with boys, who treated her badly but gave her attention she craved. She also began to experiment with drugs.

> I was in the eighth grade when boys showed interest in me, and I craved the attention so I played along, pretending I liked how they talked to or treated me, but I knew something was wrong. I knew that people were talking about me at school, because popular boys who never spoke to me before were trying to come on to me, and they would tell me what others were saying about my reputation. I was angry inside, but I felt I had no one to talk to, no one to trust; and what would they do about it anyway. I was trapped. I also tried alcohol and marijuana for the first time; I wanted to see what it was all about.

In high school, Haley became a heavy drug user, which brought her trouble with authorities and did nothing to stem the abuse she received from peers or lessen her painful isolation.

> As I begun high school I changed, now I was back to being a little fish in a big pond, and I

tried different groups to try to fit in. Eventually, I ended up with the stoners and partiers. I was still only on the fringes of this group, and no close connections with anybody. The only thing we had in common is that they too had trouble fitting in and we were all in trouble with the school, grades, detention. I experimented with every drug I could. I used pot every day, and always had it on me. I had a period of time when I was tripping on acid every other day. By that time my time in school was useless. I was not doing any work, and socially withdrawn from everyone. It was a blur, until I met some friends outside of school who partied on the weekends at raves and rolled on ecstasy. I guess I was still going to school on the weekdays because I got arrested for acid in my Junior year and was eventually kicked out for something I did while being severely bullied by a group of classmates. I thought my life was over.

At 18, Haley's mother was diagnosed with breast cancer. During her mother's health crisis, Halley felt overwhelmed. She tried to get help, but was refused care, and then attempted suicide.

My mother was diagnosed with breast cancer, and I ran away for the night. I knew I needed mental/medical help but was refused by a facility. My parents picked me up the next day and I went home to kill myself. Being unsuccessful I was in the hospital for a week because of an overdose, then transported to an inpatient facility for a month.

Haley entered into treatment and was given medication for depression and bipolar syndrome but remained a heavy street drug user.

> I finally felt that I was being taken care of for my problems and started antidepressants and was no longer suicidal. When I got out of the hospital I went back to old friends and some drugs, but I had changed.

At the same time, Haley's mother went into remission but continued to smoke and drink heavily. An attempt at family counseling failed, with the mother bitterly saying that it had been used as an excuse to "blame me for everything."

Haley writes,

> For the next few years, I spent time in relationships and moved around a lot with the boyfriends. I enjoyed the travelling and doing new things, but was still smoking pot, depressed, lonely and felt unfulfilled.

Haley's painful isolation, years of being abused and treated as a sexual object caused her to become jaded. Her feelings that there was no one who cared for her or could help her caused her to become nihilistic and she was attracted to Satanism. Despite this, Haley's feelings of hopelessness and loneliness caused her to strongly desire a community to provide her with love and attention.

While still living with a drug-addicted boyfriend, Haley attended a fundamentalist revival meeting and asked for deliverance from addictions. In answer to her sudden prayer, Haley received miraculous immediate healing of her addictive behavior. Grateful, she joined the very conservative religious church as a zealot.

> I received Christ at a church which changed the way I viewed life; I quit drugs and alcohol the day of conversion and I started attending Bible teaching churches and followed their directions of what was "good" so I wouldn't go to hell or fall back into drug addiction.
>
> They told me I had a new family with brothers and sisters by my side. They really cared about me and I wasn't so lonely anymore. I felt reborn.
>
> It was suggested that I follow everything they told me to do and not to do.

Psychosis

> Early in my experience, a woman approached me who had been off her psychotropic medications because people told her they were 'evil' and that I should do the same; and that God would heal me of my depression and bi-polar disorder. Since God had delivered me from years of drug addiction, I thoroughly believed God would heal my mental illness. Beginning at that time, I began to go on and off medications. Due to the inability to remain stable at

my full time job doing clerical work, I would start up again.

My behavior drastically changed because I was trying to be holy and never sin. After two years at the job, I quit my position because my dreams of becoming an African missionary evolved into a six week expedition, therefore I quit my job before travelling and on my way to Africa I flushed all my meds, 'once and for all.' I promised to God I would never take those 'evil drugs' again.

Haley committed to a life of service, including rebuilding homes in Central American after a hurricane and working with AIDS orphans in Africa. Her religious devotion was an expression of her gratitude for the very real salvation from drugs and dysfunction that she had been given.

The next couple years that followed, my religious rituals intensified. Some of these rituals included dedicated Bible reading, attending every Bible study I could, praying and fasting very often, and disassociating with anyone I considered evil, including my parents. This seemed to be the best way to show my devotion to God, and it seemed that God was doing miracles on my behalf. After reading sections of Scripture, I would experience something similar to what I had read. I would also try to reenact some of the stories. When fasting came up in the readings, I would fast for days at a time, sometimes even without water. I began to lose weight; something I have always struggled with. When this happened, I became anorexic; and delusions, hallucinations and extreme paranoia developed. I thought that everything that happened around me was to show the evil in things, so that I would avoid those activities or thoughts. Every thought I had, I believed God was talking to me and I would even hear audible commands to do things such as walk up to strangers and tell them about God and ask them if they know Jesus. People were very standoffish, especially because I was becoming emaciated.

I felt that I was a prophet from God, a holy and anointed person that God called to save his people and cause them to turn from their evil ways. I often acted out scenes in the bible that the prophets did, including praying for rain such as Elisha did when there was a drought. Or that God had me in the 'desert' of emotion just as the Israelites did when they were disobedient to God. I felt the pain of David in the Psalms and felt that suffering was devotion to God. I felt I was different because God called me to be holy and that everyone else who did not follow the bible was going to go to hell.

Every scripture in the Bible had special power to fight of demons and evil spirits. I would stay up all night until the early morning warding off and fighting evil spirits by yelling out Bible verses or reading entire books of the Bible out loud. Such as; 'Get behind me Satan,' or 'Jesus is Lord,' or 'The Blood of Christ,' or just 'JESUS!' These were all sayings that I used to repel demons and very strong beliefs of condemnation and hallucinations that the presence of these beings were over powering and that I could not sleep or rest because they would take over my body and take me to hell. That I could die and not be considered saved.

I supposed that I knew that these were strange ideas yet I was rebelling against society at large and wanted to be extreme so I would make an impact and a statement. I felt that my part of being holy would change the world or at least scare them into feeling guilty about their sins. I knew that spending weeks and months alone in my room, when my roommate was having a party and that I would not come out because I was writing down scriptures on loose leaf paper that I put in huge binders was not healthy; and when no one was looking, I stole a piece of cheesecake which was totally against my diet regimen. My daily diet at that time was; one egg in the morning (cooked with butter only), a handful of almonds and a carrot or two for an afternoon snack. Sometimes I would make a batch of brown rice with peas and carrots in it, or a big pot of boiled beans for a treat. I felt that bland was acceptable, because anything that tasted good was unholy and I was paranoid to take that chance.

...the people in the church and the preachers would always give extreme examples of people who were condemned to hell and what they did to 'deserve' it. Week after week and Bible study after study; I heard how bad I was and began to beat myself to death trying to be a 'good' person. I stopped watching any form of TV during this time, which lasted 4 or 5 years (including movies); because the media was evil, according to the church community I was involved in.

...I began to fear that everything was evil and that I was going to hell if I did not behave correctly, which included my daily activities, such as eating and bathing. So, I would stand at the kitchen counter for most of the day reading the Bible and when I was tempted to eat or take medicine I would wait for a sign or a Bible verse to tell me it was ok to do these things. I had a duffle bag packed by the door just in case God told me to fly to Africa again.

Even inanimate objects usually held evil characteristics and I became extremely fearful of everything including; food, household decorations, such as ceramic animals and figurines, money, pretty clothes, makeup and jewelry, other books and religions.

> I began to wear only donated, outdated clothing because I felt vanity was evil. I did not care for my hygiene or cut my hair. I usually did not go to the bathroom because I felt it was weak to relieve myself. I would not wear warm clothing in cold weather and sometimes slept on the hard tile to prove I was not comforting my physical or emotional self. I felt through self-denial was the way to spiritual blessings. I figured that if I died trying to be holy, I would go straight to heaven.

Meanwhile, the health of Haley's mother worsened, with the cancer returning. She was given only a couple years to live, and began a slow decline that was mirrored by her daughter's decompensating.

In response to her mother's health, Haley sought to save her both by encouraging her mother to give up her addictions and to accept Jesus. The mother and father remained unaffected, and saw Haley's behavior as an annoyance.

> I was committed to a mental hospital a couple times during this period. On my first trip to the mental hospital I still refused to take medicine, and I did not eat appropriately until I was threatened with the hospital inserting a feeding tube into my stomach unless I ate food. They released me after a week due to my rejection of treatment. Yet, while I was there, I was holding Bible studies and praying with all the patients; because of course, I thought the hospital was persecuting the Christians.

Finally, on the second trip, where I was almost homeless, having serious delusions and still rejecting medications, my father came to visit me and said he had some bad news. I asked him, 'What hospital is Mom in?' He was shocked that I knew before he told me that she was in the hospital. I assumed that she was sick because when she visited me for the last time before she died, she looked very weak. Yet, I found it very interesting I knew the truth of the situation. Also, I called an acquaintance on the phone from the hospital, who was an old co-worker; she was travelling for her employer and had a weight problem. I smelled the aroma of chocolate and asked her blamefully, 'Have you been eating a lot of chocolate?' She said that, yes, she had been and felt bad about herself.

When almost everyone had abandoned the idea that I was ever going to get well, my old neighbor and close family friend decided to visit me in the hospital. I told her I was reading the Bible right before she got there and that it said I should fast for three more days, and she got so upset she was about to leave; and I felt if I did not take the medicine that I was a lost case. So, I began taking the medication. I approached the front desk of the nurses' station and asked for my medicine, but I was also about to take a bite of an apple, and I felt that it was obviously a symbol that I was being deceived by 'the serpent' in the Garden of Eden, just as Eve had when she ate the Fruit of the Tree of Life. This went on and on and on for a long time.

During this time, Haley's mother passed on from her cancer, with Haley deeply psychotic and anorexic, seeking to be an example. Her church community believed that her mother had been condemned and in aftermath of mother's death, unable to bear the judgment her church laid on her mom, Haley left the church and returned to heavy partying. She writes,

> The pendulum swung so far to the other extreme many months later and I abandoned the God thing, convinced that I was doomed, and tried to escape the madness and started taking drugs and living on the streets in my car. Eventually, landing in jail for a month and a half and finally getting sober in AA and back on track.

Post-psychosis

Haley's diagnosis was switched to schizoaffective and she now uses a cocktail of medication.

> Medication compliance is the main course of action for me against becoming psychotic, which would happen very quickly without it. I know several friends with the disease of bipolar and scitzo-effective disorder and often episodes do occur and hospitalization is often needed. Apparently, drug and alcohol addic-

> tion plays a huge role in illness and as a mentally ill person.
>
> I have tried to self-medicate with alcohol and drugs for many, many years; which, exasperates the hallucinations and delusions. I found for myself and many others, that self-help groups and group therapy has been highly effective for discussing symptoms and problems associated with mental illness. The camaraderie of fellow sufferers is very safe and helps with the feeling of isolation and stigmatism decrease. Intensive one on one therapy with a psychologist and medication management with a psychiatrist is also paramount.
>
> ...it will be six years since then [the arrest] and it's been an uphill climb, yet very much worth it.

As she has continued, Haley has explored spirituality that is more liberal and developed maturity in her relationships with others. She has returned to college and plans to become a counselor after she graduates.

Despite the hardships of her life, Haley frequently expresses gratitude and faith.

> I realized that I am capable to anything I put my mind to; also, that I am a strong person. Yet, I believe that I can share these experiences with others that have delusions and hallucinations and tell them there is hope beyond illness....

Thank you for giving me the chance to share my story and experiences in the hope it will raise awareness in those who are suffering and those that suffer with them. There IS hope, and NEVER give up! There are others who face these difficulties and you are never alone.

In this journey, psychosis was an expression of larger movement from being a young woman lost in drug addiction and nihilism through reaction as a fundamentalist into devout but spiritually liberal person in dual recovery. Haley's belief in miracles was based on her real life experience of immediate deliverance from heavy drug use and dysfunctional relationships during her first attendance of a religious revival meeting. Haley's highly religious fundamentalism represented exaggerated and symbolic attempts to transform her personal world and save herself and her mother from family dysfunction

MIKE

Discovering sacred feminine mysteries

Mike, a man who was in our schizophrenic peer recovery group in the 1990s, describes his journey through psychosis as an awakening of his inner sensitive nature that had been buried under layers of trauma. He writes of his journey from a sensitive child who underwent trauma in his family and school life, struggled with a personality bordering on being anti-social, and a journey beginning during psychosis of discovering the traditional feminine world he was denied growing up.

Personal world

Mike indicates that he was a sensitive child, recalling events like laying on a harden bank of drifted snow as a young child, looking for ten to twenty minutes at the deep blue winter sky and appreciating its beauty. He also recalled writing about Eider Ducks for a third grade writing project and being so taken with the beauty of the animals that he wrote "eating these ducks is cannibalism," a statement that would be echoed a few years later when he became a vegetarian around his fifteenth birthday.

Despite Mike's gentleness, he grew up in a family with intergenerational abuse on both sides and a severe gender bias favoring men in both the men and women of the family. Mike's maternal grandmother exhibited narcissism and emotional abusiveness, yet frequently expressed adoration of her son, who grew into adulthood as a severely abusive, racist and alcoholic man. The grandmother denigrated her daughters, feeling that they could never measure up to being as good as a man. Mike's paternal grandfather was also abusive, who became a sober alcoholic that was described as "tyrant" by one family member. Mike identified his own father as narcissistic and emotionally abusive, with his mother alternating between being dependent and meek and angry and conflicting with the father. He writes,

> During my childhood, I understood nothing about the family patterns that were affecting me. The history of family abuse, the favoring of men over women by everyone and the affect it was having on my family was all buried. All I knew was that when I was very young, some of my first memories included my father yell-

ing at my Mom while tears were streaming down her face, and, later, that my parents argued all the time.

Mike's two older brothers were also angry. After moving to a small town, Mike and one brother were singled out for their lack of religious beliefs.

> My family moved to a conservative religious town and we were raised without religion and we believed in things like evolution, racial tolerance and long hair on men being acceptable. After the kids found out I didn't believe that god existed, they gathered around me like I was a leper and told me I was going to hell. It was very frightening. This went on for as long as I had contact with these people. In retrospect, I realized it was a way for a clique of rich kids to pick on me—the rich kids picked on other kids for other things, like not being smart or being heavy, but at the time I didn't realize it was just part of the rich clique picking on everyone.

> After moving to this new town and being singled out for near-daily emotional abuse, I remember lying in bed at night, hearing my parents argue, and thinking that I was living in a cursed house.

When Mike was ten, he was molested by one of his brothers, and after about a year he suppressed the memory.

> I guess it was too painful to handle and I more-or-less forgot about it. But it made me

very angry, though I didn't realize it at the time. I began to think in very violent ways and I wrote some very disturbed fiction, like about this terrible fictional world controlled by a totalitarian government where the rebels—the 'good guys'—were cannibals.

With this internal world, I was developing a very angry inner self and began to have a bad temper. I didn't get along with many people and I also had a strong lack of perception—I would miss obvious hints, nonverbal communication and would never be able to recognize when girls were showing interest in me. I would need clear statements said directly to me to understand anything and this resulted in several times when I was very insensitive and hurtful without recognizing or intending consciously to be so. I think some people, especially girls, thought I was an insensitive jerk, and I don't know if that was something I unconsciously intended or if I wanted so much not to be where I was that I was just totally unaware of the world around me.

When I was in seventh grade my parents divorced and my Dad lived in a nearby apartment. I was often left to visit him and he would be gone for hours. I explored the apartment and found sadistic porn books. As it turned out, he was having a sick sexual relationship with the wife of another man.

That summer my parents attempted to reconcile with my Dad living with us again but them not married. After a few weeks, they began to argue a lot. By late July, they were screaming at each other all day, every day. My family had three birthdays in August and they screamed at each other all throughout August. My Dad's birthday came and went, and they screamed at each other all day long; my birthday came and went and they kept screaming; one of my brothers birthday came and went nearly two weeks later and they still were screaming all day every day.

Finally, it got quiet but still it was very tense. My brothers and I were all walking on eggshells. After a few days, our parents gathered us together and told us they had decided to remarry. This was miserable news for us; virtually the only thing worse they could have told us is that they were going to die.

In early high school things began to change—my Mom and brothers were leaving for college and house was quieting down. I had started to hang out with a liberal group of church youth in a nearby city, while still being an atheist—and I read Thoreau and Gandhi and converted to pacifism and vegetarianism without knowing anyone who was either one. In retrospect, I was reacting to my inner rage. I really didn't know what it meant to be a pacifist and so I really didn't change inside. Instead, this created a charming exterior with my anger seething inside. I expressed this anger by being very competitive intellectually and arguing with people a lot. I was always trying to prove I was right about everything. I got quite clever at sounding smart and as far as I was concerned I was always right, so I was very arrogant and would look down at people as stupid.

Mike began adulthood with narrow focus on career and failed to make lasting relationships with others, especially girlfriends. He went to college with an ambition to have a successful academic career, resulting in him moving out of state to attend a university with an intensive honors program. Mike's parents divorced during this time. He experienced a separation from his mother, who had been attending a university two hours away getting an advance degree during his high school years. Meanwhile, Mike had a close though emotionally cold relationship with his father, who could be charming.

Soon after going to the college with the intensive program, Mike faced a personal crisis.

> After a year in one college, I transferred to a big university out of state, and I became promiscuous. At the end of my first year there I met a woman who I impregnated. She was from a very sexist country and had been horribly abused growing up and was disowned by her family for dating me.
>
> Though she and I didn't know each other that well, she and I wanted to keep the child. I told

my father I wanted to marry the woman and keep the child to 'do right' by her, but he disagreed and we argued for months, with my father insisting on an abortion.

The woman and I married, but I immediately got cold feet. My family was mad at me for marrying her, my then-wife and I felt grief-stricken about the abortion, and we were under a lot of pressure. I was very angry at everything and I began to severely misperceive things and I was to mean to her, oftentimes without knowing it. She responded by being subservient and sexually manipulative, and we fell into a cycle where I kept getting meaner and she became more and more subservient and manipulative. It was during this time that I recalled being molested by my brother for the first time in years.

After about nine months of marriage, I told her that I was thinking we should probably break up, she became very angry and we fought continually. We began to sleep apart as a sort of separation, but we couldn't afford to live separately. She was also mean by now, and would try to make me mad by flirting with other men, saying mean things to me in front of friends, and so on—when she is angry, she will try to make the other person very angry.

Psychosis

A year after being married, I left our trailer after an argument with my then-wife and three voices exploded in my head, two women and one man, arguing with each other. I didn't recognize any of the voices as my own. After the storm of voices stopped yelling at each other, I realized that something was wrong and I needed help.

I decided to seek help from 35 year old feminist woman in my graduate department, where I had been admitted while still finishing my undergraduate work. It was obvious that my marriage was a huge problem in my life and I needed to find someone to talk to about it. I began to approach this older woman, getting to know her so I could feel safe in confiding in her and I began to open up to her.

About this time my ex-wife confronted me on how mean I had been to her, which I hadn't recognized until then, and I crashed into deep regret. My ex-wife's temper really began to come out and she threw heavy mug at my head. I went to live in my graduate office on campus.

I told the older woman about this and she sent me to counseling and also suggested I do group counseling with a self-help group in the area. I began to experience voices, strange smells, and all the while I was becoming aware of personal and family patterns that were causing this crisis with my ex-wife. All the history of abuse in the family, how angry my father had always been, him yelling at my Mom while she cried, I began to understand all of that and how my marriage was continuing these family patterns.

I became interested in tarot and mysticism, after life-long atheism. I felt I could sense spiritual energy and had many unusual experiences mixed with the insights I was having. Soon after I began counseling I 'remembered' again about being molested and for the first time clearly recognized it as significant.

At this time, I was coming back from visiting with the older graduate student and her friends and I saw a rainbow between me and them. I took it as a sign that they had angelic energy that they were sending into the world and I could trust them. It seemed like they could lead me to a new life.

Because I was separated from my ex-wife, I calmed down that summer and the strange events, the voices and smells, stopped. In the fall, I began the self-help group to work on personal and life issues and I gave up professional counseling. But, because I hadn't done my graduate work, my graduate appointment was suspended and I had to return to home to live with my ex-wife.

Pretty soon, things flared up with my ex-wife again, the game playing and anger continued on both our parts and the strange events returned. I gave my ex-wife several thousand dollars from a student loan so she could get her own apartment. All the while I confided my troubles to older friends who tried to help me with my personal issues.

Crises continued with my ex-wife and I was unable to focus on my graduate thesis. During a visit to my home town my ex-wife moved in with friend of mine from junior high. My old friend had hallmarks of being abuser and I received messages from strange events and coincidences saying he would beat her. I tried to warn her but she saw it as me trying to interfere with her life. The abuse did happen several years later and continued on and off for years.

Inside I was seething about everything wrong in the world and all around me, but while I tried to put together my college career I was attracting numerous coeds, especially some very forward third world women. It seemed like some possible relationships would likely to lead to relationship like my ex-wife's, with servitude and sexual manipulation as part of the deal. I would rant about the evils of world, but I felt tempted to return to a relationship with a subservient third world woman.

During this time I had a series of hallucinations with god and Jesus. I thought Jesus was saying I was going to be condemned for being a horrible sinner. I began to hallucinate a lot and became very delusional. I saw person who looked like he was all ashen cinders, like he was in hell, and I freaked out. Friends call my Mom and she came and took me home. I was suicidal and after a few weeks I voluntarily went to a mental hospital. I believed I should kill myself and I was condemned.

I spilled my guts to intake people about all my issues and nothing I said was ever mentioned again. I was given very superficial attention and told 'take this pill and everything will be fine'.

I spent a year in and out of mental hospitals, believing I was condemned for eternity. I stopped telling people what I thought and was experiencing because they held it against me and nurses and aides would report what I said to the doctors.

I was about to return to college, still very delusional. I called old friends and asked them about a very important event that had happened during a group counseling session. I found out that no one remembered the events at all the way I did, so it began to dawn on me that maybe I wasn't going to hell.

When I returned to college, I no longer believed that I was condemned but I still wasn't taking medication. I continued to have problems and was unable to do my studies. I misperceived people and things, becoming more delusional and hearing voices.

At the same time, I envisioned 'discovering sacred feminine mysteries' as I way for me to magically transform the world so it world overcome sexism. This started in conversations I had with the older feminist friend and with my frequent reading of a recently created tarot deck called 'MotherPeace Tarot'. The images and philosophy in the deck and accompanying books were very important to me and helped me understand my personal world and the importance of respecting traditional feminine traits like sensitivity, compassion, creativity and nurturing.

During this time I told my mother I had been molested by one of my brothers. I returned home and told my mother everything wrong I'd ever done. I was still delusional and I wrote a letter to my older feminist friend saying 'The television told me to kill myself but the sun gave me a reprieve.' When I visited the friend a month later, she used the word 'hallucination' for the first time for what I was experiencing—I immediately decided to take medication from that point forward.

Post-psychosis

At that point I stabilized. I stopped hearing and seeing things, finished my college degrees and began my career. I spent years trying to improve myself, to lessen my anger and align myself with my ideals. I used neo-pagan religious rituals to cleanse myself of anger and I began years of exploring neo-pagan and new age Feminist theology trying to understand the feminine. I spent about ten years without a date, but I had a lot of friendships with women so I could get their perspectives and try to understand what they wanted and needed.

I finally met an independent-minded woman with a strong desire for a traditional family arrangement without patriarchal domination. She loves crafts, homemaking and family dinners and at the same time feels free about telling me what she thinks and what's right and wrong—including with me. She is strong-willed and intolerant of meanness in men, including in those who treat me badly.

As I committed to having a long-term relationship with her, I had personal crisis where I was more-or-less asked by events to either commit to being the person I had become or to backslide into the person I had been. I finally confronted the men in my immediate family, writing them angry letters about their abuse, including about being molested. I broke off contact with everyone in my family except my mother. This allowed me to cement my new personality into who I really am.

To Mike's painful surprise, the attempt to speak out on the abuse in the family led to a backlash from his original family.

After several months of silence, my old family tried to set up a family conference with an old psychiatrist of mine to 'get his medication corrected.' I was deeply confused and hurt by this at the time, but I now see this as another betrayal by my family trying to hide from the shame of incest and abuse by identifying me and my schizophrenia as the problem.

Eventually, Mike and his new partner married, living separate from the men in his original family and enjoying life with a blended family that includes her adult children from a previous marriage, much less anger and much more harmony than what he grew up with.

My wife and I have a very happy life because we have managed to make real the ideals I discovered in psychosis. The events in psychosis were expression of my life situation and contained important lessons which I misperceived as applying to everyone. By sorting out meaningful from random events I was able to become who I needed to be a good and happy person.

Mike expresses lasting pain at

... having an original family that does not love me or really care for the sort of person I am.

They would rather have me as I was—a person who was seething with anger—than to show a normal amount of concern and compassion for me as an incest survivor and schizophrenic.

I try not to dwell on it, but in writing this a lot of painful memories came up. I struggle with bitterness toward my original family and with feelings of betrayal. I really don't understand how they can look themselves in the mirror every morning and not feel remorse for what they've done. I struggle with occasional flashbacks of my old, angry self, mainly in the form of internalized rage and bitterness. For a while I talked to my counselor, my wife and my mom about having a group counseling session with my family to reconcile the past, but all three of them said my father and the brother who molested me aren't interested in any sort of reconciliation. Now that my mom's passed on, if it wasn't for my new family I would be all alone in this world.

As I recognize this again and again, I am more and more grateful to my wife and her family. I feel blessed to be in my new family and share the joy of a family that loves each other. I am grateful for having gone through psychosis, which showed me my spiritual challenges and helped me find a solution. I am grateful to

> many good people who stood by me—ranging from my mother to friends to professionals—and helped me become someone who could care for a family and appreciate the love they give in return.

Shortly after writing this, the brother who had molested Mike contacted him over email. Mike replied that if the brother wanted contact with him he needed to apologize for molesting him. To Mike's great surprise, the brother did so after 40 years of silence about the abuse. Mike began tentative attempts to communicate with his brother in a meaningful way about their lives together.

At the time of publication of this book, Mike reported that after a single, brief letter his brother had broken off the exchange. Mike indicated that he had been forgiving and compassionate in his letters to his brother, including having his counselor review Mike's letters prior to sending them. Mike said that in the response, Mike's brother indicated that he "had moved on from mistakes" he made when he and Mike were younger. From this Mike gained the impression that his brother had instances of consensual homosexual activities when he was an adolescent and young man and that his brother did not clearly differentiate between his molesting Mike and these other, consensual, events. Mike's brother had not contacted Mike in six months, which Mike welcomed.

> I wanted to give him one more chance to reconcile with me. It is clear he doesn't want to do this. Like my father, now that he knows that I am ready to discuss our family life honestly, he will only contact me when it is absolutely

necessary. I am certain they have no idea the harm they did or are they concerned about it as someone with a normal conscience would be. I am glad that I am a schizophrenic, because otherwise I might have ended up like them.

Mike's father has remained emotionally abusive. To protect himself, Mike has not spoken to his father for over a year and a half, though they exchange greeting cards during holidays and birthdays. The remaining members of his family have passed on. Meanwhile, Mike continues to enjoy his life with his wife and chosen family.

In this journey, Mike's psychotic reaction to his family's history of abuse and sexism led him to envision discovering the "secrets of the sacred feminine" and save the world in doing so. This vision was made concrete by completing his emotional and personal development to the degree that Mike is a happy family man and a responsible and loving partner to his new wife. Following the pattern of having a vision for the entire world actually apply to the personal world, seeking a "Golden Age of the Sacred Feminine" for the larger world actually manifested in a happy life for him with his chosen family.

WILL

Precognition leads into "delusional" religion

In a post-psychotic survey, Will, a man gifted with heightened intuition/psychic abilities recounted his journey from being confused and disturbed by his insights to seeing them as a gift. As such, his journey through psychosis included an unfolding of his spiritual self into a religion and philosophy that allowed him to use his gifts as an integrated part of his life.

Personal world

I was about eight years old when my family moved to [city and state deleted], into an old farmhouse whose construction dated back before the revolutionary war. It was a beautiful old colonial with six fire places, and eleven large rooms--five of which were bedrooms. It was here, in this setting, where I first started to experience early symptoms of schizophrenia.

Around seventh grade, I began to have sensations that someone was touching me and I began to hear voices. We now know these are tactile and auditory hallucinations caused by my unique brain chemistry, but back then Mom and Dad had absolutely no inkling of what it was or any understanding of mental illness. Since we lived in an old, spooky colonial farmhouse, it was easier for my family to think the house was haunted than to think what their son was experiencing was the start of a severe mental illness--schizophrenia.

Mom thought herself a good Catholic and asked a priest to come and bless the house. This did little for me, but it did set off an argument between Mom and Dad. The unending argument made me feel worse, because I thought I was the cause of the tension between them. To add to my troubles, my brothers teased me about what I was saying. They didn't understand how absolutely real this all was.

This was the most terrifying time in my illness because I was scared out of my mind that external forces--ghosts or even worse, demons-- were the cause of my experiences. In my innocence, these beliefs caused me to desperately cling to the tenets of Christianity. I bought into the 'ballyhoo' that God and Jesus are able to solve everyone's problems. But there was no relief from the prayers of a young man whose symptoms were now manifesting themselves at school. The unanswered prayers continuously caused me to doubt the existence of God. Why wasn't he helping me? What had I done so he would hate me? Why was this all happening to me? All these were the questions of a young boy experiencing what couldn't be explained.

Whether because of the possible expense or potential for shame, my parents never did take me to a psychiatrist. So for years unbeknownst to our neighbors, Mom's priest or Dad's congregational minister continued to bless our house and sometimes blessed me as an afterthought. It was not until high school that I shared the goings on with my paternal grandmother and found some relief by changing the way I framed what was happening to me.

Native Americans have a different view of my experience. Their spiritual perspective is that these symptoms are manifestations of a Shaman, a Native American Holy man. For me this was a much better 'deal' than thinking demons were tormenting me for un-confessed sin. So I swapped out my beliefs for a Shamanistic explanation in which I had a special and privileged connection to the universe. The reduction in my stress and nervousness was profound, because by that singular choice I changed my perspective from one of the tormented to the triumphant.

After this change in thinking, I became super successful. My grades improved, I enlisted in the Air Force, and when I came back I was employed as a machinist at Electric Boat and saved money which I invested into real estate. After a time, my net worth grew to equal a million dollars. Almost everything I was involved in yielded prosperity. Life was good, but then three events happened that caused me to reassess my view of the universe and my place in it.

The first event was the death of my daughter, [name deleted]. On a visit to her maternal grandmother, she pulled out of her mom's hand and ran into the road and was killed instantly by a car. In my grief, I also felt extremely guilty because my relationship with her mom never developed. I regret not being there for my child. But her mom and I were too young, and also her family didn't think I was an appropriate choice for her partner. They meddled in the relationship, and she sided with her parents. I was so hurt that I don't think I even shared the news of my daughter's birth with my family. I did get to see, hold, play and love [name deleted], and when she died so suddenly and so young, I was tormented by all the 'what ifs' and they tore me up inside.

The second event was that the wife I had married didn't take well to learning of the existence of another child outside of our marriage. She let me know she had been having an on and off affair with a guy, and used my grief about [daughter's name deleted] as an excuse to leave me. So she left, taking our daughter, [second daughter's name deleted], with her adding to my despair in losing those I loved.

The third event was the death of my brother [name deleted] when he died in a car accident. [Brother's name deleted] and I were very close growing up. An accident is not really an accurate description of what happened as [name deleted] was run off the road by a Navy person in a drug deal gone bad, and who instead of taking responsibility, drove off into the night. My brother was pronounced dead on arrival at the hospital and the individual responsible was later caught and sued in civil court.

Psychosis

While I use the term "psychosis," Will emphasizes that his beliefs and experiences were based on legitimate and meaningful events that are simply misunderstood by our society. As such, he remains adamant that these experiences do not need to cause dysfunction or be categorized as delusional.

> These three stressors, tightly packed into a short time cause me to 'pop my paranoia cork.' I began to think God and the universe were out to get me. My voices, that in my shamanistic beliefs were special and helpful, became overwhelming and derogatory. The gentle touches became punches to the head and body. For relief, I yelled back at the torment which scared folks in public and who called the police. I was arrested many times, and I eventually was involuntarily committed to [name deleted] State Hospital. Every bad thing that happened only provided evidence that I was correct in my belief that God and the universe were persecuting me.
>
> Indeed, bad things continued to happen. Because of my mental illness, my family took control of my property and belongings. There was a fire in my house, and my father and brothers did not use the insurance money to repair it fully. My father lost all my money

and property in a botched real-estate deal meant to help him pursue his dream of owning a restaurant. I cycled between hospitalization, prison, and homelessness. I lost everything as a consequence of schizophrenia. Neither my Shamanistic beliefs nor Christianity were of any comfort now. I longed for spiritual knowledge and understanding. I read the Bible, Books on Wicca, The Koran, The Book of Mormon, The Satanic Bible, the History of Religion, Quantum Psychics and meta-psychics, anything I could get my hands on to gain any sense of my relationship to the universe.

I read all these books because I needed to come to terms with my precognition; premonitions about the future which usually come true. When I was Christian my church called it prophecy when I held Native American beliefs my grandmother called me 'Obomsawin' (oh-bohm-sah-ween) an Eastern Pequot/Abenaki word roughly translated as 'the one who leads.' A psychiatrist once tried to convince me that my precognition was 'psychosis' a symptom of schizophrenia. I told him his wife would have a car accident and she did within two days. He immediately called the police accusing me of setting it up. The police investigated the incident and were satisfied I had no part in it. My precognition is random, it's always a little unsettling when it happens, and regrettably I can't pick the lottery numbers.

In the hospital, psychiatrists were telling me that I'd be in the hospital the rest of my life, and indeed at that time there were people there who had been there for thirty and forty years. The doctors said I'd never be employed; I'd never have a family, and that this was the fate of a person with schizophrenia. Then the State of [name deleted] decided, because of the failing economy, to close the State Hospital. I was discharged into homelessness.

While homeless and living under a bridge in back of a soup kitchen, some people came to my isolated campsite to smoke crack. I was naïve about drugs. They handed me a loaded glass stem, and I took my first hit of cocaine. BANG! From that point on, for eight years, I was addicted to crack cocaine. And for eight years, all my time was spent in drug seeking behavior. It was one of the most difficult things to lay-down and the process was not linear. I 'slipped and fell' many times until I got it right. Even now, after nearly fifteen years clean, I still have 'coke dreams' when I get stressed.

During one of my hospitalizations, a woman named Yvette Sangster came to the ward and did a presentation on a recovery and advocacy program she was directing. She said things in direct opposition to what the psychiatrists were telling me. She said that schizophrenia was not a fate to be surrendered to, but an illness that could be managed and recovered from. She said to find out what I needed to do to get better and to do those things. This changed my life. I was back in control of my destiny and that I could learn my way back to sanity, community and my family.

I took Yvette's advocacy class and eventually became one of her best advocates. The personal empowerment I learned also allowed me to reevaluate my spiritual beliefs. I was no longer the victim of circumstances; I was no longer floating helplessly in a universe or mental health system that I could not influence. I put a positive spin on all the bad things that had happened to me. I now viewed schizophrenia as a useful journey to enlightenment. I 'dumped all the junk' in my belief system that did not work. I no longer believed in an invisible man or woman in the sky, who wanted to burn me in hell, who needed my money and who I could manipulate with prayer to change the universe in my favor.

In Will's post-psychotic survey, he also discussed his exploration of his abilities and attempts to find a spiritual tradition he could identify with. While his therapists attempted to minimize his precognition and explain it in mundane ways, Will sought out those who would accept magical and mystical thinking.

I at one time attended a fundamentalist church who 'laid on hands' to heal me of my schizophrenia. They convinced me to go off all medication as a sign of my faith; proof that I accepted the healing. It ended badly with me needing to be hospitalized. More to the point of this question of experiential delusions, I experienced people exercising their faith by speaking in tongues (glossolalia).

After those experiences my voices (auditory hallucinations) mimicked what I had heard and practiced in church. This caused me to think I was having some kind of spiritual or supernatural experience.

My fellow church goers encouraged me to stand up for my faith and prompted me to speak in tongues in front of my psychiatrist; who immediately hospitalized me coercing large increases in medication. He was absolutely flabbergasted that members of my faith community who visited me practiced glossolalia as part of their spiritual lives. He did everything he could to band them from the hospital.

Later, the man joined a highly mystical spiritual group that encouraged trance states, use of oracles and beliefs in thought manifestation, including successful individual and group magical rituals. In discussing this new spiritual group, he wrote,

> Interestingly enough there are others who believe in precognition not as a symptom but as a gift. I hooked up with those folks, it might make me feel much, much better. Also, as I mentioned there are folks who believe in precognition but my condition of afore-knowledge came first then I started looking into the phenomena and people who are like minded.

Will wrote in his survey that his mystical beliefs matched his experiences, which he affirmed by saying

> I do believe in magic. I think everyone believes in magic at some deep level; it's part of our sociology, culture and history. In retrospect I have sought out [mystical spirituality] because in searching for meaning for what I was experiencing, the definition of magic kept popping up. Others told me I was magical out of which evolved thinking myself magical, having had precognitive events that I could not explain with psychiatry or medical science. I can't recall having a preconception about magic other than a child's fantasy in fairy tale books.

> In the medical world precognition is labeled psychosis in [my spirituality] it's labeled gifted. One man's trash is another man's treasure. I was having experiences that I didn't have an explanation for in the belief system forced on me by my parents. My belief system now matches my life's experiences and I feel a lot less stress. I fit in, in this belief system whereas I did not fit in, in the Judeo-Christian

belief system. Just this adaptation has made it possible to focus on recovery and spirituality in many other ways.

... did I just learn to say something different or actually set aside the belief is the question. Am I saying the same things only to different people? I would say I have not set aside the beliefs others labeled as delusions but only learned to express myself differently. Who is to judge really? If you believe in angels you would have to admit that the possibility exists that in the myriad sea of DNA diversity, world population Six billion, nine hundred fifty four million, seven hundred fourteen thousand five hundred seventy four someone just might have the ability to listen to them. Catholics think so and some are called saints. Is there precognition? Millions think so. Can I believe in my ability to help others experience recovery and advocate for a recovery orientated mental health system as a quest and that spiritual concepts play a part in how I live my life? Absolutely I hope everyone would.

For me, hallucinations are different than delusions. I see movement in piles of rocks or leaves and the movement burst forth with creatures. Very scary! Even through medicated I still see the movement but through years therapy I have learned coping skills and react differently. Realizing I'm seeing something that someone else can't see is a mechanism of

> social cues. Or even the odd question, 'do you see that?' I now do my sculpture of the bugs and scary stuff to take control over them. Others now see them too [smile]."

During the survey review process, evaluators, including professionals, who had no knowledge of Will, indicated he appeared psychotic based on the content of his essay.

Post-psychosis

> I became very eclectic, and kept bits and pieces of belief systems that worked—such as the concept that we should treat others the same way that we would like to be treated. Wiccan, Christianity, Judaism, Buddhism, Atheism, all became just 'menus of ideas' that I could pick from to gather items that worked for me.
>
> My journey led me to realize that spirituality is a concept that can benefit others and should not be used as a self-serving tool to try bend the forces of nature to help us out when we do not like the circumstances of our lives. My journey has led me to an exceptional life. My symptoms no longer control me nor does religion or fear of the unknown. I live in a suburban community with a loving wife. I am employed in a great job in which I can help those just like me. I advocate for recovery oriented systems of care, and I take care of my health-- physical, mental, and spiritual. No matter why I was born or how long I have to live, or why

> I'm here, I enjoy my life and that perhaps is the most important spiritual lesson of all.

At this time Will takes medication to control hallucinations and occasional anxiety.

> Even today, in stressful situations all my hallucinations (visual, auditory, tactile) increase. As matter of practice, I practice self-help stress techniques. However, on [date deleted] a tornado by chance blew over my house and my neighborhood causing much damage. Some nut tourist touring the damage area said that, 'God punished the wicked here with the tornado.' For some unknown reason his statement stuck in my head as an unwanted thought as if I was supposed to be punished because I had damage to my property. The stress of that statement even though bizarre caused my symptoms to worsen and I needed to resort to Xanax for a couple of weeks.

Regarding his work, Will wrote in his post-psychotic survey,

> My Quest then is to get through this life without destroying myself and in the process perhaps doing something extraordinary. Can I achieve something great? You bet I can and I believe we all have the potential of doing something great. Now that I'm less worried (and less criticized) that my mental health differences are problematic; in my mental health systems advocacy I can help people like me. I

can help people with mental illness by advocating for a recovery orientated system of care.

Is my quest successful or am I effective? That may be judged somewhere down the line. I think I am affecting the [state name deleted] Mental Health System and even [organization name deleted] in small ways that down the road will make a big difference. If I think of advocacy as small effects on an asteroid far away; changing the course only by a smidgeon of a degree will in the long term (a billon miles) will result in a great distance from the original destination. Missing earth as an example.

Some folks are distinguished by making the big splash; an event that changes everything, i.e. a big lawsuit or a big change in policy. Most of us advocates are stuck in making the small differences, setting up the possibility for a large change. I am proud to be one of the advocates who were able to get the [state name deleted] Mental Health System's Commissioner [name deleted] to come out with [policy/program name deleted]. That recovery shall be the overarching goal of the state mental health system. Recovery from mental illness was once thought to be delusional, now it's reality. Can advocates do the same here in [different state name deleted]? We think so, and we hope so!

Shortly after completing survey, Will was recognized nationally for his work in promoting peer recovery. He currently is the Executive Director of a state peer organization and works with dedication and passion to aid the recovery of others. Given his personal and professional success, I believe there is ample evidence that Will is an effective advocate for recovery and when survey evaluators indicated they believed he was psychotic they were unable to understand Will's life from biased and narrow secular and medical viewpoints.

JOHN

Self-discovery as a mystical artist

In his journey, John underwent two periods of psychosis during and immediately after his college career. It is particularly notable in that his episodes were comparatively brief and his relationships of trust allowed him to come to understand his condition much more quickly than many.

In addition to these aspects of his journey, John underwent comparatively low amounts of trauma in his life, both from the perspective of outsiders and from his own perceptions. This indicates that his psychosis may not have been a result of trauma, but something that occurred for other reasons. Three possibilities in particular seem to be likely factors in the development of his psychosis: (1) the existence of mental illness in a grandmother; (2) a wistful desire, after initial experimentation with LSD, to "go crazy" to explore the deeper aspects of life; and (3) an inner drive to merge his Christian identity with his artistic and hip inner self, leading to his new vision of the role of Christ Consciousness in the modern age.

Personal world

John had a fairly happy childhood in Christian home and, unlike many teenagers raised as Christians, identified as a Christian into his young adolescence. His parents remain married until early adulthood, but divorced after several years of tension. The father remarried soon after divorce and there was the possibility of a long-standing, secret affair. Even so, John's personal world was marked by low level of trauma and the dysfunction he encountered was within normal range for mainstream society.

Though having a happy childhood, John writes that his grandmother had died from mental illness.

> My grandmother once tried to commit herself to a mental hospital. When the doctors asked her if she ever thought of killing herself, she replied that she could never do something that horrible to her grandchildren. And so the doctors sent her home. One week later, the F.B.I men came for her and she leaped from a sky view apartment story window, one sunny afternoon when I was five years old and playing tag, when my mother called us into the house to explain that Grandma was so sick that she made herself die.

As a young man, John went to college to become journalist and was assigned to be art critic in the college newspaper. Despite being artistic, John was not studying or creating art and he was severely criticized in college art community as critic who did not understand art.

Around the same time John experimented with drugs, including marijuana and LSD, which he found exhilarating, and after initial experiences with LSD, he wistfully wished to "go crazy" as way to explore deeper aspects of life.

Psychosis

John's reviews in the student newspaper continued to draw sharp criticism and this caused a great deal of stress.

> My first serious break was triggered by stress. I had involved myself in many activities related to school and the building of a career, pushed myself in journalism at the student newspaper. My role as an art critic brought criticism from the arts community, which greatly stressed me as I am an artist in my own mind, and the complaints stemmed officially from my lack of a traditional actual artist background, but I think really came from my own mind becoming psychotic and not able to relate those thoughts to a more sane world, so I now see the controversy as really an affliction of insanism, which I define as extreme prejudice akin to hate from the sane community because they don't see the world as we do. I really wanted to prove myself as a writer and as an artistically minded person, but pretty much went down in flames.
>
> My delusions involved the government hunting me, being famous for hideous crimes, and

the world wanting to kill me, delusions that probably literally resulted from getting criticized on an art review that described artwork in an insane light. Now I find this hysterically funny, as the best art is insane, that's the whole point, and if you need an art background in order to appreciate the art then the art has failed.

During this time, the John believed that he was continuously being filmed and events were being staged to make him commit suicide on camera as an example to others. Feeling overwhelmed and surrounded, he took an overdose of sleeping pills in front of his college roommate, who immediately called 911. John writes,

> A couple of months before [the suicide attempt], the voices had told me they were there, charging into my head one night as I lay in bed. They drooled and paced like dogs. They were going to get me, they said. No matter what I did, they were going to tear me limb from limb until I acknowledged they were infinite in the universe.
>
> In just two weeks before I swallowed the pills, my life had spiraled out of control. I was a sophomore in college three weeks into spring quarter and had been hearing voices for months. In the past week and a half before swallowing the pills, I hadn't been to class once, not out of laziness, but out of genuine fear. In one particular class I managed to struggle my way into in spite of the voices, the

professor eavesdropped my thoughts, picked each one up out of its cage and sent it scurrying into the underbrush. He could read me, and I am sure he was telling the FBI just what I thought of their wing tip shoes and gray unassuming Chevrolets. That professor was crazy, his scatter brain sizzled out his ears from too much acid he ate in college, and his warped thinking wanted to consume mine.

Or it appeared so at the time.

As days progressed my brain wouldn't stop tripping. Twisted ideas had taken over my head. People were out to get me. The university was hunting me down for my liberal ideas and I was pretty sure the F.B.I. was somehow involved, listening on my phone, tapping my dorm room and following me where ever I went with an invisible movie camera, recording every event of my day and broadcasting it on Public Television.

Four days before I swallowed the pills, I knew something was desperately wrong and I sought professional help, going down to the university clinic. I stood in line, was handed a card to check the box that best explained my symptoms. There was a box for allergies. There was a box for vomiting. There was even a box for dizziness or nausea. But there was no box for being hunted by the F.B.I. and I couldn't explain to anyone what was happening to me. All I knew was that it scared me white, and their blank stares would never help. I bolted out the door with cameras on my back and people whispering orders in the bushes.

I feared for my family's safety, because who knows when this conspiracy would get them too? All hints in conversation pertained to killing me or my family. The jig was up, and I was already too late.

Coming home to kill himself, John writes,

> [Friend's name deleted] was on the couch. He had been talking to emergency officials, he had been biding his time, trying to offer me some way out of whatever was happening to me. He said he didn't know where to go, or what to do. We were just living and life would go on. Wouldn't I please just let it?
>
> In my desk I found a half package of sleeping pills I had bought to get some peace and sense. In front of [friend's name deleted], I swallowed the handful to fix my head, fix me good and make all of this go away.
>
> I realize now that I didn't take the pills as some kind of death wish. I wanted to live, but I was drowning and the pills were my scream.
>
> If I wanted to die, I would have swallowed the pills in secret, not while my friend sat watching me on the couch. I overdosed on pills and put my friend at the controls. [Friend's name

deleted] was immediately on the phone, telling them I was ready.

John was taken by ambulance to the hospital where his stomach was pumped. The next day his mother came and had an ambulance take him to a mental hospital near their home four hours away. Both John's mother and father visited him, expressing love for him, gratitude that he was alive and encouraging him to look positively at life.

> For a good two weeks after the slip, I was deluded that the world hated me. Friends, professors, the world at large wanted me dead, hated me for failing them, for going down. I stayed stuck in my head, afraid of my debt to society, until one day [friend's name deleted] walked into my room right out of the sky, arms open like he was catching the world. He and two friends had driven the five-hour drive from [city deleted] to the hospital I stayed at in [city deleted], just to see me. Right then everything turned completely around, and I let go of the bottom and headed towards the light. My debt had been forgiven. All that mattered was healing.

John credited group therapy with helping him manage his experiences.

> In group, we learned tricks to understand ourselves, how some thoughts hurt, but weren't necessarily valid or true. We learned to break thoughts down and digest them for what they were. We learned to free ourselves from the

really nasty thoughts. We carved our delusions back into the form of reality and released the crazy birds locked in our minds.

The patients helped each other just as much as the doctors. We encouraged each other in the daily circles, stretched our limbs and thoughts and began to feel good again. My real healing began when I helped others to heal.

[Name deleted], just a shade younger than me, was crippled by his own mind. He came in a wheel chair and he didn't move. His mother sat by him at the breakfast table and nursed French toast into his mouth, wiping his chin as the syrup dribbled down. The man had haunted eyes, frozen in ice by staring at the Devil, and his muscles were locked up. For the first few days, he didn't scratch, stretch or yawn. He just sat there like a piece of furniture, and his mother would talk to him like she was talking to herself, wiping his mouth as he stared empty into space.

And then one day while I was reading *Calvin and Hobbes* on a couch, he spoke to me. 'Friends are good,' he said. I nodded. He moved for the first time in days. He relaxed in that wheelchair, and he even smiled. Soon I brought him to my room and fed him Easter chocolate that I was learning how to taste again, and he became my best friend in that hospital. He stood up from the wheel chair without a scratch. Two nights later, we hosted a Caddy Shack movie night on the ward. We shared pot-smoking stories, almost as if we had ourselves a joint to pass, and laughed at the stoner antics of Bill Murray and Chevy Chase. We had a bond beyond group therapy. We laughed.

Helping him out of that wheel chair helped me out of my hole.

After my first break, it took me some time, perhaps months, to realize the full extent of my delusions. Some delusional beliefs, such as the idea that the university controlled me and I was on TV, lasted a good three or four months after hospitalization and medication stabilization.

In discussing his rapid return to good health, John writes,

> I experimented with LSD before my brain sprouted into a hallucinogen. I was curious. Mind enhancement was on the rise. I was at an age where everything seemed wonderfully possible, and acid taught appreciation of possibility, a sense of magic beneath the body of things.
>
> For the first few times, acid is a hot air balloon ride, seeing the world from a different stoop riding a cloud. The first spins of acid are fun and games, riddles for enlightenment. You learn to think new thoughts in new ways. The

sun struts happy and you go swimming in the sky.

But do it often enough, and dark questions will unwind from the shadows. You never know what you may find inside your head, what demons will seep out of the cracks of everything you were once sure of. Getting burned is part of the learning process. Skin heals, and the Universe carries on.

The tricks of LSD and the symptoms of schizophrenia are virtually identical—heavy hallucinations, delusional thought, sensation of riding the drama of the Cosmos. But LSD wears off in eight hours. Schizophrenia doesn't stop until something stops you.

Like acid, the beginning of schizophrenia is a trip. I was onto something, following down a line nobody else saw, sure it led to salvation, a deeper understanding of everything I had once took for granted. I had an energy no one else connected with, an energy that was going to make me great. I was bouncing, wandering the streets with a musical wisdom in my head, buzzing on the wings of angelic butterflies, fantasizing babbling spinning patterns like a spider's web.

But follow that connection long enough, and the sky will break and spiral down to hell. Every schizophrenic trips a bad trip because the spinning will consume like a nightmare she completely believes in, and the worst atrocities she can imagine become real for consumption.

The acid culture taught me how to heal and grow from nightmare. The acid culture was a circus of thought, a Dr. Seuessed conception of music and light inspired through temporary, drug-induced schizophrenia. Acid mystified insanity. Instead of a drooling mess in a straitjacket, insanity can be a divine clown juggling knives on a unicycle with big red shoes.

Rather than a horribly traumatic collapse best medicated and forgotten about, my psychotic attacks were remarkable learning experiences, shocked glimpses beyond time of my place above and beyond this body. I looked my demon in the eye, and I woke in the arms of my creator.

Bad dreams filter blood, prove how deeply a brain can imagine.

In the haze of my last hospitalization, I amazed doctors by how fast I came back. They had expected ten days before I would be ready for sunlight again. Within five days, my mind had made its scabs and was ready to be released.

The soul can sprout wings and fly again.

I learned how to heal by watching acid casualties heal. Bad trips learned how to come back one day at a time, taking the nightmare into perspective and learning the world all over again. They would never be the same, but they would be wiser and stronger for the travel.

Even an awful experience can teach great wonder.

After stabilization, John returned to college and completed his degree, ready to begin his adult life. However, with the excitement of the time John decompensated. His experiences were marked by a coincidence with a hitchhiking musician from a different state but a city with the same name as John's college town.

> I stopped for these two hitchhikers, shadows of lightning in the pouring rain, and they threw their packs and one guitar into my trunk and we were headed down the highway with the slosh of the rain. The one in back quickly fell into himself and went to sleep, while the one in front relaxed on a cigarette, leaned into the seat and shared a conversation.
>
> They were on the Further Tour of 1998, The Other Ones (what was left of the Grateful Dead) with Rusted Root and Hot Tuna.
>
> The man was named Leaf, and he had 'Live Free' tattooed in bare-knuckle statements. When I mentioned [John's college town deleted] as my destination, his eyes lit up. They were from [city with same name as John's college town and different state deleted] and were on their way there in time. He was a musician traveling for songs, picking up songs

like change in a hat down a musical road in the tradition of Woody Guthrie.

Sloppy sleep in his eyes, the man stated that he needed to drop his mother a line; he called her periodically to tell her he was all right. He was wondering around the countryside, and for all I knew he could quite literally have been an angel.

Their exit came and I left them at the freeway just above where they were going, south to [state deleted] and the alternative [city deleted]. I traveled west, in the rain and the haze of dream music, and flopped into [John's college town deleted] on a friend's couch about two in the morning.

The next night, we were summer slouching, hanging off a porch with a few beers, a bellyful of food and a freedom in the air. [Friend's name deleted] talked about her trip last spring, the couches she slept on, the people she met, the stories that unwound at her feet and from the pile on her lap. And she talked of this musician who gave her a couch to sleep on and a pillow to catch the dreams.

He fed her songs, orange juice and a glimpse of [same city and different state deleted] style. He was a story and a glimpse, and she passed him by in the night on the way down the road.

And his name was Leaf, a name that stuck in my mind in a blur of an echo.

'Did he have 'Live Free' written in his knuckles?' I asked.

She said, 'Yeah,' her mind open like a question mark, 'how did you know?'

That porch breathed a numbing hum trembling through me. She had met the same kid 5,000/??? miles away, five months before hand, and told his name in a conversation the very night after I had met the same kid, 5,0000?, having randomly picked him up in the flashing rain, and everything fit together as moments happen like Dominoes. It was an astounding coincidence, given about the same odds as the exact same person being born twice.

But there is a drummer to the rhythm, and nothing is an accident that wasn't meant to happen. Things carry themselves, in a perfect order, like water rolling down a leaf.

I was filled with a wonder that a sense of intelligence infinitely magical was behind everything, whispering to me, telling me voices like thoughts wondering out loud. Leaf popped in and out of my life at that moment for very good reasons – to show me the world was magical.

Three days later and I was back at the mental hospital.

On the second breakdown, which wasn't so much stress induced, aside from just having graduated college as a major life changing event, I was on a quest to save the world. I thought I was Christ, I was going to lead followers and travel around and turn them on through poetry. Again, the earlier Leaf story helped to confirm the Christ thought, and I've always had a heightened spiritual understanding, believing I was talking directly to God in a regular conversation starting at the age of 12. I felt I was at least a prophet, and that the world was ending, and I must be there to save it.

At the time of my second psychosis, Camel cigarettes had just been banned from using Joe Camel in advertising, and switched to driving a billboard truck advertising Camels through a family neighborhood. In my delusion, I equated the truck with the Devil, and felt that I was on a quest to stop it.

I called my mother in the middle of the night from a payphone after being lost in rural Ohio to tell her I was going to visit my dead grandparents. She told me I as hallucinating and needed to get to a hospital.

I eventually came into contact with police officers and was taken into custody, went through a psychotic hellish experience where I feared, imagined psychotically experienced raping crucifixion, and that miracle coincidence [with Leaf] appeared in my mind as proof of an intelligent magic beyond the simple laws of probability, almost like God looking me in the face of the mystical. After getting released from the mental hospital, I go for a walk by myself, and then randomly encounter "Leaf" spray painted in graffiti on the doorway. All three instances of Leaf were witnessed by non-psychotic people, as my friend confirmed the tattoo that I quoted word for word, and the graffiti was on the building for some time after my psychosis had receded, and was also witnessed by non-psychotic people.

Post-psychosis

Once again, John was able to return to stability quickly. In reflecting on his life, John writes,

> I am schizophrenic. I think tied-died, stretchy thoughts, see through kaleidoscoped eyes, and keenly feel that shock of life that pumps blood, inhales wind and dreams when the moon is watching, the essence that flows without knowing how and simply is.
>
> I sip life dwelling in the gardens of very good people, but I was dragged through the ends of hell to get here. I faced amputation, torture, being buried alive. I stared demons square in their Adam's apples, believed completely in nightmares and monsters, and walked to the other side.
>
> But schizophrenia is no curse. It blesses my vision, shows me there is mystery beneath the numbers, enigma behind everything we think we know for sure, and awakens me to a curi-

ous wonder of things as simple as a raindrop sliding down a leaf. I learned to be amazed by simple things like clouds and grass, and am absolutely astonished how everyday things can even be possible. Schizophrenia taught me secrets of the universe through question marks.

After his passage through psychosis, John found work with a newspaper in his college town and was chosen to be a columnist for a hip, artistic, younger person's section of the paper. John became prominent as hip journalist and performance artist poet through his work, receiving attention and appreciation from the community of young artists and bohemians.

During this time he worked on refining "Clang" poetry in which words sound like ideas being expressed. John writes,

> [T]he best art is insane, that's the whole point, and if you need an art background in order to appreciate the art then the art has failed. I now work to make art of insanity through poetry, writing a lyrical style I coin Clang, which is written using a schizophrenic interpretation of sound that reflects the psychotic experience. In this way, I am healing and putting a renewed understanding on that stress that seemed to break me in the first place.
>
> I equate my psychotic experiences to mystical experiences, and try to interpret them through

myth, as I find this to be the most healthy perspective.

I don't look at my experience with psychosis as being a negative sickness, but something that makes me different. It's very related to my identity, as I approach the world with a mystical, magical understanding. I this way my experience with psychosis has heightened me spirituality and given me an insight to reality most don't understand. My psychotic episodes help me experience the dying process, which gives me renewed inspiration and appetite for living. We are only here a short while, this world is but a dream, and we must experience it as fully as we can. I've learned that I am apart of all essence, the Is, and that understanding has greatly enriched my experience of this world.

I still carry this Christ insane thinking [the belief that he is Christ from the second psychotic break], though I've learned to relate it to reality in certain ways in order for it to match with the literal world. I believe that mankind's next step is to realize that it is part of God, akin to say the Son of God, but Christ just realized it first. In Christian myth, he is predicted to come back. I interpret that he comes back all the time in the spirit of people who openly love, which is our next state of evolution. Since love is our next state, anyone who realizes and inacts this is the son or daughter of God, hence a Christ. In truth, you can find Christ beings emerging in many forms of history. In my myth mind, I believe I am the literary poet version of Christ, sent to help people turn on to a Christ understanding of love through poetry. In this way, my Christ insane delusion can be carried out in a way that benefits me spiritually, mixes enough with literal reality and encourages me to be kind.

My psychosis has also given me insight and a poetic vision, which feeds my poetry and allows me to approach the muse with fresh eyes and insight. I consider my experience with schizophrenia to be a gift as well as a blessing, and I would not give it up for the world.

[The events surrounding John meeting Leaf] ...helped me realize that the delusions held some sort of truth, although spelled out in a mythical reality that collided with literal reality. I view the medication as a way of being able to keep them separate. It's not that the meds make me less crazy, but teach me to keep the crazy myths separate from literal reality, serve to keep me centered in the world's reality time zone. I view the described coincidence as a miracle that proves the relevance of mysticism, and my whole psychotic experience as an early triggered death experience, showing me mystical truths that most people don't realize until they've stepped into the door out of this world, into the beyond.

As years have passed John continues to use marijuana and anti-psychotic medication, though a doctor prescribing the medication has indicated that were he to stop using marijuana he might be able to stop using the anti-psychotics. He has spent more than a decade in full employment, is married, and is currently supporting his wife in her graduate schoolwork. At the time of this writing John's wife had just given birth to their first child.

Now in a very urban setting, John enjoys creating performance art poetry at an urban poetry happening near a subway stop in arts area of city. A square is chalked off and artists are given two minutes to perform their art, helping him further refine his poetry to make it succinct and powerfully concise.

John remains on good terms with both his father and mother and others in family, probably in part to the lack of abnormal family trauma and his ability to merge his childhood identity as a Christian with his hip, artistic inner self. He sees his journey through psychosis as allowing a poetic, mystical and life-affirming self to emerge that fulfills Christ Consciousness in his daily life.

THERESA

From isolation to a loving family

The journey of Theresa, documented in Paris William's *Rethinking Madness,* best exemplifies the contention that psychosis can serve the person as a catalyst that moves the person from a disharmonious web of life to a harmonious web. In the journey recounted below, psychosis creates an intuitive image of a means to "save the world" through Theresa conceiving a child.

In retrospect, Theresa sees this idea as expressing a deeply personal and suppressed desire for a fulfilling family life. Having had a childhood where she often felt lonely and isolated and an early adulthood that was marked by conflict and tragic deaths, Theresa had difficulty having relationships and had decided that she would probably never have children or marry.

Despite this conscious conviction, Theresa's unconscious desires were strongly expressed in her vision of saving the world through having a child. As Theresa tells the story, miraculous events move her through trials and dangers into an encounter that enabled her to realize her vision of saving her own personal world and creating the family she desired.

The following material is taken from Paris William's *Rethinking Madness's* chapter of Theresa's story, with sections rearranged to tell the story in chronological order. It is reprinted with the very kind permission of Paris Williams and Theresa.

Personal world

> I think I probably had a pretty cushy early few years, you know, until about four or five, and then my sister was born, and that was all okay, but I think all of a sudden, I kind of had gone from . . . . being the center of everybody's attention to kind of nobody's attention

[laughs]. In the course of a normal type of life without other kinds of things layered on top, it probably would have been nothing, but . . .it was kind of a bit of a shock, you know, sort of around the time I was starting school which is quite an intense time for little kids, anyway. So I kind of got this sense of disconnection that started right back then, you know, and then I didn't make friends particularly easily at school.

Things started falling apart with my parents' marriage [when] I was about seven or eight or something like that, and so there was a lot of conflict and . . . things just started there and just went from bad to worse with their relationship and never really recovered. . . . [Mom] took us off and [then] she was just kind of on the move. . . .I went to more schools than I could remember. [My parents] had a couple of goes at getting back together, so there was all this kind of hope and stuff when they did . . . just that sense of stability, you know, maybe it will come back, you know [laughs]. But before the boxes were unpacked, they were fighting again.

So, there was kind of just . . . layers and layers and layers of a similar kind of . . .you know, moving further and further into myself, I think, you know, and less and less able to trust what was going on around me...um...less and less able to trust them, as well. . . . A sort of a disconnection, you know . . . moving schools and not making friends, you know, and not really feeling connected to anything, you know, so . . . it's not difficult to see where those layers and things kind of come from.

Apart from those kind of early things, I mean, normally I think I probably could have survived and managed without, you know, developing psychosis . . . later on in my life, but then Mom dropped dead and pretty much just suddenly dropped dead, as well. She had a brain hemorrhage, and it was so sudden that...yeah, our life kind of changed overnight, basically. . . . I was sixteen, so I was still in school, just at the end of school . . . so we moved . . . to live with my father. . . . It was completely miserable for a couple of years until I moved out 'cause we hadn't had a huge amount of contact with him and he was living with a woman that he'd been living with for quite a long time who we didn't like, [and] she didn't particularly want us around. . . . And then four years after that, when I was twenty, dad dropped dead as well, pretty much. . . . So I think, you know, the other stuff by itself might not have needed such an outlet that was quite so extreme, you know [laughs], but the deaths and quite sudden deaths, particularly of Mom, were more than I could probably handle and not have it have to come out in some way.

> We had no grief counseling of any kind. . . . I think it wouldn't have taken much at that point, but I don't even remember anyone saying, how do you feel, you know. It sort of didn't happen, which means that everything pretty much, you know, all of those kind of layers, you know, just got pushed sort of further and further down and further and further in.
>
> So I started drinking, which was, you know, which was...fine [laughs]. . . . I mean that helped me sort of skip along the surface of those things.
>
> [I didn't feel] as important as everybody else or everything else around me.

She speaks here to her belief that perhaps one role of her psychosis was to develop that sense of self worth.

> I seemed to need to break through something to get to the point where I could sort of allow myself to...I don't know...um...to have what I needed somehow.

About a year after her father passed away, at age 21, Theresa followed her desire to travel, eventually ending up on a kibbutz in Israel. She describes the kibbutz as "a bit like my ultimate heaven."

> It was, you know, a big family feeling kind of place, communal living, kind of everything that had been missing for me for a long time.
>
> Because it was so heavenly, it kind of brought to the surface all of the kinds of things that I'd

been dealing with, or hadn't actually dealt with. . . . I was having a great time, you know, but I was drinking. I practically just wasn't sober, you know, and so I sort of understand it like, it was all there but it was too much. . . . It was overwhelming and I couldn't cope with it, so I had to kind of suppress it the best way that I could, and then it just kind of bubbled through, you know, and... and just put me over [laughs].

Psychosis

However, over time, she "decided it was actually Heaven." In time, though, the experience of being in Heaven began to alternate with powerful experiences of also being in Hell. Some experiences in the early stages of this included visual hallucinations both on the television and in the environment.

> [I saw] a lot of fiery landscape scenes, kind of classic Hell looking stuff, people transforming into demons, colors changing from normal to red and black. Normal scenes transforming into hellish looking ones. People mutating into horrible looking demonic type creatures.
>
> I was . . . doing things like climbing a high hill behind the kibbutz and working very hard in the kitchens with no breaks, etc......this seemed to be mainly about how hard I could strive.....if I could strive hard enough I could save others from hardships and protect them from having to suffer.

These feelings of compulsive heroic striving sometimes combined with the visual images of being in Hell, creating experiences in which she "would have to walk through a hell type thing, you know, like fire."

She discovered that yet another force was driving some of her experiences—a desire to have a child, a desire that she later realized was closely intertwined with her desire to have a family. Both of these desires were present prior to her psychosis, and she believes they fed directly into the more anomalous but closely related experiences that occurred during her psychosis. One particularly prominent anomalous experience related to these that arose during her time at the kibbutz was the sense that "if [she] was to have a child, it was to save the whole of humanity," though she was not consciously trying to have a child. "I actually was trying to get pregnant on the kibbutz but not consciously (i.e., was pretty promiscuous and forgetting to take the pill)."

After several months of gradually moving further and further away from consensus reality, Theresa's traveling companion became very concerned and decided to take her to a psychiatric hospital. Unfortunately, Theresa found her treatment there to be more harmful than anything she had yet experienced.

> I got immediately assessed as being deeply psychotic, and was put on heavy medication, incredibly heavy medication, that knocked me out for about three days. . . . And when I came to, I didn't really recognize myself at all, and I couldn't think, I couldn't really do anything at all, and [I had], you know, one of those zombie

kind of shuffles. . . . [I went] from someone who . . . was, you know, full of beans and had a lot of energy. It was like from one extreme to another. So the trauma of that was probably as bad as if not worse than the trauma of anything that had actually caused . . . the breakdown or whatever, in the first place, you know.

Theresa believes that even her friend had been significantly traumatized by the hospital experience. "My friend . . ., who's still my friend actually, was as traumatized by the whole hospital experience as I was, and so that's taken her a long time to work out as well."

Theresa finds it interesting to note that during her stay in the hospital, her sense of heroic striving remained to some degree, but the quality of it changed significantly, becoming more personal and more relevant to what was actually taking place in her environment.

> I had some stuff when I was in the hospital about walking through fire and having to survive from the ultimate kind of, I don't know, whatever the most ultimate thing you would have to survive from, I would have to survive from, you know. But I think that was more what was [actually] happening at the time. [Being in the hospital] was a traumatic experience, and I did need to survive [laughs].

> When I was in hospital in Israel, my friend came in to visit me and the staff was speaking to me in Hebrew, which is the language that they speak, and they were talking to me, and

> she got really, really angry at them and said, wait a minute, she can't understand Hebrew...she's from New Zealand. And they said to her, well, she's been speaking to us and understanding us in Hebrew for the last week. What do you mean, we just assumed she knew how to speak it. And that actually happened [laughs]. It's not a delusion . . . but that's one of those things that [my friend] tells people that all the time, 'cause she just thinks it's incredible, you know [laughs].

After being released from the hospital, Theresa was sent home to New Zealand, where she was nearly admitted to hospital but it was decided she could live with her Aunt, Uncle, Grandmother and their family though she remained on heavy doses of antipsychotics. About four to six months later, she moved away from her family and into her own place and completely stopped taking the antipsychotics, though did continue to struggle with difficult experiences for some time. About two years later, following a personal development course that was aimed at breaking down physical and emotional limitations, Theresa entered her second period of psychosis. In retrospect, she believes that the antipsychotics did play a major role in stopping her psychotic experiences during her first period of psychosis; however, she believes that this did not ultimately serve her well at all, since it merely interrupted a process that needed to be worked through.

> The way I understand it now is that the first [period of psychosis or transformation] kind of got interrupted, you know, with the drugs,

> with the medication, and so the whole process just got stopped, basically. What it was that I was working through and needed to work through just kind of got halted. . . . The purpose that it had, that it was serving, to work through those things that we were talking about before, the trauma and stuff, didn't have a chance to come to a natural kind of conclusion or fruition or whatever, to evolve to where it was needing to be.

About a year after returning home, during the period of time that she now believes was essentially a latency period between her two periods of psychosis, Theresa began to attend intensive personal development courses.

> They were slightly cultish really in a way that you kind of did these weekend workshops and . . . they encouraged you to kind of surround yourself with people who want you to win and all of this kind of stuff . . . and they cost thousands and thousands of dollars. . . . So I kind of got into that and then ended up becoming what I thought was quite connected to the people that were there, and I probably was, but I did isolate myself very much from anyone that wasn't involved in the courses (which they actually encouraged you to do).

Theresa recalls that a particular theme began to become more and more prominent in her consciousness during these courses, which was her desire to have a family. She recalled being surprised initially when she felt the first stirrings of this desire.

> Because I think there was kind of grief and trauma associated with it, I had decided I was never gonna have children, and [laughs] . . . on one level anyway, I sort of thought . . . I won't bother getting married and I won't have children and that kind of stuff, you know.

However, as these courses forced her to inquire more deeply into her longings and aspirations, this longing for a family became undeniable.

> [During] one of those courses, one of the early ones . . . you had to make . . . some kind of vision for your life or create some...I think you had to make a promise or something like that, and mine was something to do with having a family or creating a family.

> That was actually probably what I wanted most, but I couldn't kind of handle it, you know." Theresa believes now that, even prior to her psychosis, she may have been struggling with this core dilemma of wanting a family, yet not feeling that she could "handle it." She now believes her psychosis may have actually been playing an important developmental role in this regard. "I seemed to need to...um...break through something to get to the point where I could allow myself to have what I needed somehow. Yeah. I think...maybe I had to be psychotic to make it happen.

> The final course that I did was a weeklong intensive thing where you go off in the bush. It

was called breakthrough, break through your mental and physical limits of the things that you think are possible in your life, and that's the idea of it. So I wasn't drinking or doing anything like taking any drugs, but they did use what I now understand to be kind of like mind control techniques really, sleep deprivation and intensive physical exercise and stress and things like that, and I slipped sort of slowly into another mental crisis, I suppose you'd call it, and [soon] became what would be defined by psychiatrists probably as intensely psychotic again.

[This time,] I was actually consciously trying to get pregnant, i.e. had ideas that the creative moment would happen at a certain phase of the moon, with certain writing on the walls of my bedroom, and helped by particular crystals, etc. . . . I completely sort of graffiti'ed the inside of my flat [with] all kinds of curly things [that] artistically expressed all sorts of things to do with creation. I assumed I was kind of channeling a child [laughs]. That's what was going on in my head, you know. . . . And strangely enough, it worked – that is to say, I did get pregnant.

I had similar thoughts/feeling both times . . . that I was expanding and expansive to the point that there were no boundaries between me and the rest of the universe and . . . that I could bring about the healing of humanity by

> bringing all that is good into the spark that would create a child.
>
> The second psychosis was also similar in being about physically striving. I had a push bike which I rode all weathers – including long distances thru driving rain etc; walked and then swam out into the sea, walked long distances – aiming to find things to climb (I scaled a really high fence with razor wire on top once and got over it, but was caught by a security guard. I managed to convince him I was lost or something and he drove me home!!). The point of the climbing seemed to be to get to the highest point as then I would be able to see all that was below and take all the suffering I could see away from others.

Another less prominent but significant type of anomalous experience had to do with multiple realities. Theresa recalls occasions during both her psychosis in which "several different realities . . . [were] happening at the same time . . . [and] the boundaries weren't clear at all." She describes that this experience was particularly vivid during the process of regaining contact with consensus reality.

> The natural regaining of my 'normal' mind happened like that as well (and remember this was with no medication) . . . it was like the layers of 'other realityness' gradually peeled away to reveal a more 'grounded (or common sense of) normality' underneath and the more clearly the 'normality' came into focus the more I was able to realise what I needed, and

> needed to do - another way to describe it would be like seeing something in a very clear focus . . . so you know that it's real and then it gradually 'morphs' into another reality; as one starts to fade the other becomes clearer.

She believes that particularly profound healing took place during her second period of psychosis, culminating in a lasting transformation that has led to full recovery and a rich and fulfilling life.

> Before I slipped into, I guess, being in a state that probably people couldn't have related to me at all very easily, I decided that I was going to have a baby [laughs]. Yeah, and so I, you know, had a very brief relationship with an old school friend, and got pregnant. ...but while I was able to behave in a way that was relatively normal to outside appearances (well normal enough for someone to want to sleep with me!) what was going on inside me was quite different: moon phases, crystals, channeling and all kinds of magic.

> This was the beginning of my life really, in a way . . . because I mean that was the beginning of creating a family . . . . which is kind of where it was all heading, I think.

So, after longing for a family for so long, Theresa had finally become pregnant; however, she was also homeless and completely alone. She had just been evicted from her apartment, had spent the night in a homeless shelter, and found herself contemplating suicide.

> I was walking across Grafton bridge where people coincidentally quite often throw themselves off, and I sort of thought, okay, you know, considering what's ahead of me, and, you know, what's just happened, being dead would be easier than this. . . . But then I had that kind of thing . . . that quite a lot of people describe—well, the situation is as bad as it could possibly get, you know, the only way's up [laughs] . . . so just take the next step type of thing.
>
> I needed some help, so I went to Ward 10 of Auckland hospital . . . which was the psych ward, and tried to present myself there, tried to say, look I'm not well and need help . . . but they said, ah, well sorry, if you're well enough to tell us that there's something wrong with you, you're not unwell enough to be here type of thing.

Fortunately, she soon came across a drop-in center run by a group of psychiatric survivors; an encounter that she later came to realize represented another very important turning point in her recovery.

> I just wandered in. I was still actively psychotic (i.e. was having uncontrollable disturbing visions/thoughts...but mainly fears for my sanity, fear of being under psychic attack, etc.). I think I was beginning to regain my sanity and realize the situation I was in and was starting to recognize when I was in touch and out of touch with 'normal reality'. The place

had a self contained room – think they called it 'emergency accommodation' where I stayed for a week or so. Despite the stuff that was going on in my head, I actually felt safe there …..and in all the time I was wandering and psychotic (that time) I hadn't found anywhere I could just stop and feel safe……(which was something to do with the striving I think). If there was a point where my recovery started I guess it would have been there….I had the chance to stop and take a breath, gather my strength, and I realized Iactually had the strength to face what lay ahead……I found my own internal hero…..then funnily enough I met a real one !!

Post-psychosis

After being pregnant for about three or four months, Theresa met a man who began to look after her.

> I was, I don't know, a little bit strange and a little bit interesting (he says) and still pretty…um…still pretty mad, but he kind of took me under his wing, really, and fed me because I was pretty much homeless and pregnant, you know [laughs].

Theresa recalls that a particularly supportive aspect of this man's character was his groundedness.

> He actually seemed totally connected to the ground, and also not in even the slightest bit scary…..or like he would hurt me or try and make me do anything I didn't want to do,

> etc......I was so "tired" (in every sense of the word) by then, that at that point the ground (with him on it) started to look pretty good.

The stability and care that he provided were the final important resources that Theresa needed to integrate her psychotic experiences, return to consensus reality, and move in the direction of successfully raising a family.

> That quality of just accepting and respecting each other for who we are and how we feel/what we believe, etc., is something that has continued into our relationship and is one of the keys to our success, I think.

They remain together to this day, over 22 years later. After meeting her future husband, Theresa's psychotic experiences gradually became less and less until they completely disappeared. She then went about the business of having a "normal" life, raising a family and getting involved with her children's education, working part time as a nanny etc. While profoundly and deeply transformed by her experiences, they didn't actually play a part in her day to day life at all until she enrolled for a mental health support worker course (not really knowing at the time what was driving her to do that) and applied for a job as a "mental health consumer representative." When feeling very triggered by some of the stories she was hearing about people's experiences of being in the mental health system, she found that it was important that she continue the process of integrating her profound journey. About ten years after the second psychosis she began attending regular psychotherapy sessions and continued these for about six years and found this to be very helpful.

> I kind of lived in my head, really. I mean, I didn't really feel, you know what I mean, like I used my brain to think everything out.

She believes the psychotherapy reflected the psychotic experiences somewhat in that it helped her to develop ways to loosen her attachment to her thinking mind and balance her experience with other ways of being. But in a grounded and fully conscious way. One way has been to reconnect with her body.

> I wasn't really very connected to my body...um...so, I've done a lot of work, I mean I've been doing yoga for years and years and years now, you know, and I've done a lot of kind of work on actually . . . just feeling, you know, and expressing my feelings rather than channeling everything through my brain, you know.

> I think [art] was kind of an outlet for all the feelings I was having that I couldn't understand with my mind. Art, for me, comes from a subconscious realm, which cuts through my usual tendency to 'think' things to death.....however, there was a drive and a desperation about [my thinking] when I was psychotic – a seeking to understand. So [art] probably did help in some way. Now I've discovered that I can tap into that same creativity....and the more I do that (just relax and let it be) the more 'critical acclaim' [my art] seems to get.

She believes that the purpose of her psychosis was ultimately to transcend her isolation and inability to meet her needs.

> I mean, [the psychotic experiences] were fulfilling, helping to fulfill or drive me to fulfill needs that I've had forever. . . . We do try and meet our own needs . . . and if you've gone through quite a lot of trauma, you know, the way that you try to meet your needs couldn't come through a normal channel, you know. . . . And I think it was that interconnectedness to anybody, you know, or anything, that I was desperately craving, you know, and so [my psychosis helped me to experience] this kind of connectedness.

Closely related to her desire for connection was her desire to have a family, and she believes her psychosis played an important role in first making this need conscious and then healing and transforming her at the depth necessary to give her the necessary capacity to fulfill this desire. "I think maybe I had to be psychotic to make it happen."

Theresa believes that because of her lack of other resources, it had become necessary for her psyche to resort to such a "desperate strategy."

> All that stuff was just very buried, and, you know, I never had any grief counseling, never spoken to anyone, you know, I mean I've read a bit but not a lot really, . . . so I didn't have any kind of tools to be able to deal with any of that, so [psychosis] was . . . my own clever

> kind of tool, I think, for breaking through and dealing with it.
>
> I've been and worked with people that are intensely psychotic, and you don't have to knock them out. . . . I didn't need that, I didn't need medication at all. I don't think anyone does, actually.
>
> I have actively sought to reign in my emotional rollercoaster world a bit - that is I've sought for more of an "even keel," rather than being tossed around with the heights and depths of my feelings - I've tried to find more of a sense of peace and balance - which I definitely have....and I'd say that I don't think that would have happened without the psychosis/journey I've been on.

Another lasting benefit Theresa attributes to having come through her journey of psychosis and recovery is a sense of much greater ease within her relationships.

> [Prior to the psychosis,] my relationships operated in a very unconscious and knee jerk reaction kind of way. I felt at the mercy of other people, so for example in personal (romantic) relationships, [I] would bolt at the first sign of trouble, rather than stopping to figure out why I reacted the way I did and what my part in this is....and [I] also didn't really think I deserved to be happy. I don't really put what feels like effort into relationships now. By that, I don't feel obliged to have relationships

> or do things for people just so they will like me. I feel like a worthwhile person now so don't have to 'try hard' to be anything I'm not....I felt for a long time that I was putting ALL the effort into all my relationships and never getting anything back for myself. Now I think that was probably because I didn't think I was truly worth it.

When asked about any lasting harms she might still experience as a result of her psychosis, Theresa responded adamantly that she could not think of any. "No, nothing, nothing, nothing [laughs]. Nothing bad came from this [laughs]."

As of the writing of this book [*Rethinking Madness*], Theresa is 48 years old. She has not taken any psychiatric drugs since she was 23. She came off of antipsychotics as soon as she was able to after her first period of psychosis and avoided them completely during her second period of psychosis, though she now notes this was more out of sheer good luck...along with a measure of driving fear and mistrust. She has not had any significant psychotic experiences since recovering from her second period of psychosis (over twenty years ago now), although she has had a few relatively minor incidents of nonconsensus experiences and/or beliefs. According to the definitions used in this study, Theresa considers herself as fully recovered. She now works within the mental health field as a consumer advisor, where she offers "peer type" support to those diagnosed with psychosis and other mental disorders. She remains married to the same man who supported her in her recovery over twenty years ago, and together they have raised two children.

* * *

In this remarkable journey retold in Paris William's *Rethinking Madness*, the fulfillment of Theresa's vision of "saving the world through having a child," though initially interrupted with psychiatric treatment, was made real by her pregnancy leading to her meeting a man who she married and shares a family with, thereby "saving" her from a personal world of isolation and personal loss. Like mythological fables we have been encouraged to discount, there are magical and miraculous events, such as Theresa communicating with Hebrew-speaking hospital staff, her climbing over a high fence topped with razor wire, her wandering into a psychiatric survivors drop-in shelter while she is pregnant, psychotic and homeless and meeting the man who would care for her and become her life-long partner and father of her children.

From a secular, Western perspective, this story fails to conform to our expectations of what is mental illness and what is possible. However, from cultures that are familiar with vision quests and fulfillments of prophecy, the story represents a fulfillment of Theresa's powerful vision of attaining salvation through having a child to save the world—meaning her personal world.

If all journeys through psychosis ended like this, there would be no need for treatment of the condition. The challenge of working with visions and miraculous attainments is that while sometimes visions are fulfilled and miracles do happen, these attainments cannot be predicted, counted on in every circumstance, or forced to occur. On the other hand, finding a means to keep the person experiencing these events calm and safe while discerning the accurate aspects of the psychosis can lead not only to a successful resolution of the passage but also to a person and life transformed for the better.

SUMMARY OBSERVATIONS ABOUT THE SPIRITUAL JOURNEYS

Most of these journeys involved the person leaving a web of life that was disharmonious and creating a new identity in a web of life that was much more harmonious. In some cases, this was related to trauma, but sometimes the journey represented a positive expansion of personal potential with minimal trauma. John is the clearest example of someone experiencing positive growth from psychosis without trauma. Psychosis also frequently expressed the inner self and the journey of the person; it frequently drove the person toward a more authentic life and/or gave insights that helped transform the person's life for the better.

In all of the examples, remarkable events occurred, ranging from accurate intuitions to near miraculous life-saving coincidences. In at least three examples, psychosis led people from a state of unhappiness to a fulfilling of life. In some of these cases, psychosis helped the person to become ready for or actually find long-lasting partnerships and family.

With these observations, it can be argued that in many cases psychosis actively advanced the person's life purpose in the fullest spiritual sense. Significantly, these journeys happened in naturalistic settings either without clinical help to accomplish the journey or actually despite clinical attempts to minimize and limit events.

It is useful to imagine a two dimensional graph for people in psychosis. One dimension measures the amount of trauma a person has undergone. The other dimension measures the range in which the psychotic experiences seem nonsensical and random to a midpoint where content has been projected from the person's life to far point where the storylines parallel voluntary spiritual quests of enlightenment. In terms of trauma, Haley, Mike and Theresa have a lot of trauma, whereas John has relatively little. Will's life begins with "symptoms" which, when given proper perspective, are part of a functional and successful life until severe trauma causes a psychotic break. In terms of content, Haley and Mike mainly have projections from their lives (though both have important spiritual events), whereas Will, John and Theresa are the most like the ideal of a voluntary vision quest seeking spiritual enlightenment. The remarkable story of Theresa is like a mythic, romantic fairy tale beginning with tragic losses, proceeding through heroic striving and ending with a miraculous intervention by the Goddess of Love to save a devoted follower fallen into dire straits. In all of these journeys the person moved into a higher consciousness that allows a higher level of functioning than prior to the psychosis.

In terms of social stressors that may contribute to psychosis, experiencing isolation during an early age was reported by Haley, Mike and Theresa. On the other hand, the strength and love received by John from those around him appear crucial in his rapid recovery and his ability to use his experiences to transform his life. Haley and Mike reported early, coerced sexual encounters that led to a jaded inner self and dysfunctional, troubled relationships that contributed to significant life challenges. The deaths of loved ones were factors in the lives of Haley, Will and Theresa, with psychotic crises brought about by these deaths for Haley and Will. Given its powerful nature, any person suffering from a mental health challenge should be given special care and attention when someone they love dies.

In looking at duration and intensity of psychosis and the speed of recovery, the five stories seem to outline a general principle about the person's web of life: the ability of the person's family and peers to provide love, acceptance and compassionate emotional support prior to and during psychosis is central to recovery. The families of Haley, Mike, Will and Theresa all showed limitations in the ability to love and provide support, with Haley and Mike experiencing abuse and Theresa losing both parents while young. Will's loss of loved ones to death and divorce were key factors in his experiences becoming unmanageable. All four indicated difficulty with peers, with Haley and Mike experiencing abuse from schoolmates and Theresa experiencing isolation. Only John experienced strong family and peer support and his psychosis is noteworthy for its brevity and his ability integrate it into his life. Mike and Theresa's recoveries were aided by new friends who stood by them during the psychosis, creating a refuge that appears part of a spiritual unfolding in their lives. While receiving some support from her religious peer group, Haley, her family and the mental health system were also subject to severe judgments that weighed heavily on her and severely exacerbated her symptoms. Will's recovery appears related to personal empowerment through peer support and explorations of his spiritual gifts.

It is particularly important to note Haley, John and Theresa all sought care prior to or during severe episodes and the medical establishment either rejected them or was inadequately prepared to help them receive treatment. All three were suicidal at the time and Haley and John went on to make suicide attempts. During early psychosis, Mike turned to an acquaintance for help and eventually voluntarily entered treatment but the mental health's system refusal to help him with his serious personal problems caused him to reject medication. Will's ability to live with "symptoms" was impaired by tragic deaths and losses, resulting in forced treatment and a dual betrayal by his father stealing money that could have been used for his care and a mental health system that first locked him up and then dumped him onto the streets.

In the debate on whether or not mentally ill people are capable of insight into our condition, there is evidence here that we frequently do have insight, but our attempts to approach the mental health system are rejected, either because we are "not sick enough" to merit attention, or because our concerns are greater than simply taking a pill "to make everything better." Ironically, the medical establishment denies us treatment and ignores our legitimate issues until our condition has become so severe that we no longer understand that we are in an altered state. Given this, it appears that the medical establishment lacks as much insight into our care as we do.

Looking at stories of psychosis using the depth psychology concepts in the first passage, applying the concepts as appropriate to each story seems useful. In terms of becoming conscious of one's shadow, the story of Mike fits well.

Likewise, the unconscious coming to light is prominent in Theresa's life. As indicated earlier, reaction-formation from one way of life to another, initially through an unconscious process, is prominent parts of Haley, Mike and Theresa's journeys. In using parts of theories to help understand the experiences of people, it is important to use these concepts only as they fit the story line, rather than reading unnecessary inferences into people's lives to make them fit into an overall theory.

Intriguingly, in one post-psychotic survey, "G-10" wrote that her experiences occurred when she was studying philosophy and writing about "about being true to ourselves and about what happens when we are not true to ourselves. I[t] was about what happens to us when we experience interactions that go against who we truly are. It was about the injustice, anger, shame, and love." Her insights into the importance of being true to ourselves caused her to believe "that heaven had arrived, that I was in a reality in which everything came together and had been transformed."

In a very importance sense, the beliefs expressed by the woman are relevant and accurate here. Through the process of psychosis, people moved from a place of not being true to themselves to a place, both within and around them, where they were much more true to their inner self. They were able to make their lives much better and, metaphorically speaking, some arrived at a heavenly web of life that provides sanctuary within the hard world we all share. The writing about the importance of being true to oneself and heaven on Earth are central to this process and it is no small matter that the woman who experienced these insights had her writings destroyed by others because they deemed the insights delusional.

It is also important to recognize that all of the stories include intuitive and mystical events. Given the commonality of the events, it can and should be argued that counselors who refuse to recognize the validity of these experiences have secular biases that interfere with working with people in psychosis. The Western secular counseling perspective that refuses to acknowledge valid spiritual events like those described in these stories lessens the ability of counselors to effectively work with people in psychosis. This is especially true in the case of Will, who found that limited views of his abilities and experiences in both Western counseling and traditional religious perspectives significantly worsened his functionality, whereas an eclectic crosscultural view of spirituality allows him to be a high achiever professionally and happy personally.

While psychosis is marked by exaggerated and mistaken mystical thinking, acknowledging the validity of these events in general and using a Cognitive Behavior Therapy (CBT)-like approach to help the person in psychosis separate the valid intuitive and mystical events and insights from the false conclusions we tend to jump to can help the person (and the counselor) find a middle ground between narrow secular ignorance and grandiose, exaggerated mystical thinking.

The third passage seeks to outline an overall approach to working with people in psychosis that identifies meaning while also moving them toward stability. With the ultimate goal of helping the person both recover and transform their lives, the combined toolkit that follows seeks to recognize both the risks and the value of the unrecognized vision quest we call psychosis.

A Combined Toolkit Approach to Psychosis

THE MEDICATION DEBATE

At present, there is a very contentious debate on the utility of medication for treating psychosis with what will hopefully soon be an acknowledged common ground. The medication debate, ongoing for decades among some peers and practitioners, has a group of progressive advocates urging that medication be seen as largely counter-productive if not outright toxic to the health of people in psychosis.

The most well-known of this group is Robert Whitaker, who wrote *Mad in America* and *Anatomy of an Epidemic*, in which he contends that medication is counter-productive, unnecessary and oftentimes toxic to the person taking it. Even so, on the www.madinamerica.com web journal Whitaker has indicated that a process seeking "optimal use of medicine" is the best approach, thereby allowing that some medication use is beneficial in some circumstances. Another writer, Paris Williams, cites numerous studies of medicine use in his work, *Rethinking Madness*, indicating that long-term use of medicine to treat psychosis results in substantially worse recovery rates than not using medication. While advocating that individuals experiencing psychosis be given places of respite and care to allow the condition to run its course, Williams indicates that studies are showing the short term use of medicine is more effective than not using medicine.

Long-time peer advocate and innovator Ron Coleman of the United Kingdom's Hearing Voices Network sees psychosis as an adaptive response to trauma and has outlined a process to work with voices as a means to make the experience positive. A married family man who travels the world in his training and advocacy work, Coleman still hears voices but uses them for his benefit. In *Recovery: An Alien Concept*, Coleman makes the point that studies show that medication and other treatments forced onto people do not work in many cases. In *Working with Voices*, however, Coleman and his co-author Mike Smith recognize medicine as one response to dealing with voices and madness.

Significantly, many progressives advocate the use of Open Dialogue therapy to help work with the person in psychosis and her or his significant others. While this treatment protocol from Northern Finland uses extensive individual and group counseling to reunite the experiences and thoughts of the person with those around him or her, the treatment team also uses medication for about 20% of the people they work with.[3]

Among conservatives in the debate, E. Fuller Torrey of the Treatment Advocacy Center and author of the well-known guide *Surviving Schizophrenia*, wrote a highly critical review "Anatomy of An Epidemic – How Robert Whita-

---

[3] http://www.tandfonline.com/doi/abs/10.1080/10503300500268490#.Up4406Mo6Uk, p. 220

ker Got it Wrong" in which he strongly defended medication as being crucial to many people's recovery and not a danger to health.[4] Even so, the stalwart advocate for forced treatment and other mainstays of the medical model wrote in the review

> It has been known for a century that approximately one-quarter of individuals who develop a schizophrenia-like psychosis will recover without treatment and not get sick again. (p. 3)

Torrey then cites several studies going back as far as 70 years ago, indicating that approximately one out of four people who develop psychosis recover without long-term use of medication.Torrey concludes his highly critical review with this conciliatory statement:

> *Anatomy of an Epidemic* is not without merit, however. In addition to detailing the many wrongs of American psychiatry, it reminds us what good psychiatric practice should be regarding the use of antipsychotic drugs. Use them in as low a dose as possible for no longer as necessary. Patients with a first episode of psychosis should be taken off the drugs several months after they go into remission to ascertain whether they are among the subgroup of patients who will not need maintenance medication. As patients age their medication can

---

[4] http://www.treatmentadvocacycenter.org/home-page/71-featured-articles/2084-anatomy-of-a-non-epidemic-how-robert-whitaker-got-it-wrong

often be reduced and sometimes discontinued. (p. 8)

Given the coalescence of the medication debate, it is possible to arrive at a common ground statement, which, while probably not agreed to by most of the people cited above, does seem to me to provide a basis for compromise. This common ground can be summarized as follows:

- Medicine is not always needed and not always needed for the long term.
- If symptoms remain, medication use in the short term may be beneficial.
- Long-term medication use is best avoided if possible.
- Medication does not work in all cases.
- Pharmaceutical companies lobbying, advertising and selective support of research findings have overemphasized the effectiveness and need for medication.
- Acknowledged conservatives in medication debate are, compared to common practices in real life, much less supportive of medication use – Generally speaking, most practitioners are seen as excessive in how much and how often they prescribe medicine.

With Robert Whitaker's presentation at the annual convention of the formerly conservative National Alliance on Mental Illness (NAMI) in 2013 and the response by medical experts in modifying their always-use-and-stay-on-medication stances, progressives may feel that they are winning the debate. There is, however, a very practical difficulty with any non-medical approach to psychosis. None of the progressives are putting forward alternatives that are available in most of the United States. Approaches such as Open Dialogue, Soteria House and Hearing Voices groups are actually quite rare in the United States and it will be years before the approaches are available in any useful amount.

Fortunately, there are numerous tools that peers and family members have developed over the past two or three decades, along with some input from academics and professionals, that are available in the United States. Training for many of these approaches are available in various locations. By combining these approaches, a solid means to help a person in psychosis can be outlined and those interested in implementing the combined toolkit protocol can get all the required training within a year's time.

BUILDING EFFECTIVE TREATMENT

Approaches which seek to help those in psychosis need to account for variations in both the need for and responsiveness to medication. After years of debate and discussion, the long-standing "Typology of Three" appears to still be an accurate summary: Sometimes medicine is not needed; sometimes medicine is needed and is effective; and sometimes medicine is ineffective. A treatment plan not only needs to recognize these differences between people; it also needs to have an approach which faces the reality that when a person in psychosis enters into treatment no one knows which of these three categories the person will fall into. In short, initial treatment must be flexible enough to accommodate for all possibilities until an individualized treatment plan can be determined.

In addition to Typology of Three, the phenomenological experience of the person in psychosis is very important in outlining a treatment methodology. From a psychiatric standpoint, there is little differentiation between types of psychosis, but treatment approaches that take into account what the person is actually experiencing are central to strategies for resolution. For those whose hallucinations only include disembodied voices, one set of treatment options apply; for those who experience combinations of visual, auditory, olfactory and other hallucinations, a second set of options apply and for those who experience delusional thinking but do not experience hallucinations a third set applies. In cases where a person is only experiencing disembodied voices, such as Ron Coleman and Eleanor Longden of the Hearing Voices Network, the ability of the person to identify their personal experiences as separate from consensus experiences is much easier than those who, like I, experienced seamless combinations of hallucinations and voices. Likewise, while voices may be dialogued with effectively, images and non-reoccurring full hallucinatory experiences are much more difficult to understand. Hallucinations and voices or hallucinations alone, especially when involving events that are initially seamless (i.e., indistinguishable from consensus reality), also results in a substantially longer period of development of misperception and delusion, resulting in a tenacity of delusional beliefs and in highly confused states requiring long-term post-psychotic review to re-orient a person to his/her personal history.

On the other hand, when someone experiences delusions only—such as during group delusional psychoses or in highly excited states—the delusional aspects may lack the tenacity of delusional beliefs based on hallucinations and/or voices. In these cases, the delusional and symbolic beliefs may be more easily deciphered for their meaningful but exaggerated content that is relevant to one's life. These insights may include recognizing small group patterns that instill the beliefs and one's personal insights that were exaggerated by the exhilaration of the experience.

An example of this is in the case of G-10, who believed we were in heaven and an essential aspect of this was every person being able to be true to his or her self. As indicated before, this "delusional" belief/insight of G-10 summarizes the goal of many people's spiritual journeys and the rewards of striving to accomplish our journey, whether we have experienced psychosis or not. While experiencing sleeplessness and exhilaration during this time, G-10's insights are relevant to the journeys of the second passage and have a solid basis in a metaphorical and spiritual view of our lives.

Insofar as the Typology of Three goes, it appears to me that we are at the beginning stages of outlining approaches for all three instances. The work of Paris Williams, among others, seems helpful for those who do not require medication; the methodology of the Hearing Voices Network, in particular, Ron Coleman's work, appears to be the starting place for helping those who are not helped by medication. Meanwhile, the combined toolkit outlined below seeks to provide a means to work with people who may be helped by medication, while leaving the door open to these other, parallel, approaches.

DETAILS OF THE COMBINED TOOLKIT APPROACH

To understand the approach used by the combined toolkit, it is important to touch on the aspects of psychosis that cause people who experience it to cling to our delusions and experiences, despite the confusion and damage it causes. First, it is important to recognize that real events, some very unusual and mystical, often support the delusional framework. This was seen in several of the spiritual journeys in the second passage and ranged from a miraculous healing from addictions to a meaningful coincidence that helped the person gave the person spiritual insight and envision a new way of life. Secondly, symbolic ideas and hallucinations that are confused with literal reality can contain the seeds of much needed personal transformation, such as in the case of Mike and Theresa. Finally, the process of psychosis itself can help the person transform himself or herself and move from an unhappy, disharmonious web of life into a much more harmonious and personally meaningful web of life.

Given these observations, the goal of "treating" psychosis is to aid the person's transformational journey while enabling them to distinguish personal reality events from universal consensus reality events—in other words, know she or he is hallucinating and help him or her recognize the personal meaning contained within the experiences. In doing so, we can help people recover and transform as needed, not simply as people who are challenged by an unrecognized vision quest but also as spiritual beings who are learning our unique and crucial life lessons.

This approach has several stages towards this goal.

- Calm the person, build trust and stabilize his or her day-to-day life.
- Help the person understand the difference between personal and consensus events.
- Help the person develop a strategy to deal with their non-consensus events.
- Seek to diminish the non-consensus events so they stop entirely or are voluntary, sought after and recognized as personal events.
- Help the person gain insight to connect between personal events and his or her life.
- Help the person implement a transformation of his or her life to actualize the lessons of the experiences as part of a self-actualization of her or his spiritual being.

The main tools used in this approach include several techniques developed in recent decades by peers and family members. In combining these and other tools, it is important to see all of the tools as components to be used in whatever combination as best fits the individual situation.

The tools are:

- *Schizophrenia: A Blueprint for Recovery* by Milt Greek, a person with schizophrenia
- *Working with Voices,* by Ron Coleman, a peer, and Mike Smith

- *Personal Medicine,* part of the CommonGround software, created by Pat Deegan, a peer
- LEAP, created by Xavier Amador, a family member
- Wellness Recovery Action Plan (WRAP), created by Mary Ellen Copeland, a peer
- The process of creating an agreed-upon vocabulary from Open Dialogue, created by Jaakko Seikkula

Though most of the individuals cited above have Ph. D.'s, most of their insights stems from their lived experiences.

TREATMENT PROTOCOL TO MOVE FROM PSYCHOSIS TO STABILIZATION

Initial work

The first step for outsiders to work with a person in psychosis is to simply become familiar with the person, showing interest in them and working to build trust. This process is described in the second chapter of *Schizophrenia: A Blueprint for Recovery* and is discussed below in the section on working relationships with the person. If at all possible, during the initial period the environment around the individual should be moved towards being peaceful and positive, as outlined in the second chapter. While this initial contact and attempts at building trust is made, it is also important for the counselors and peer specialists on the treatment team to discover life content about the person through individual interviews with family members, friends and others.

It is important that these interviews be conducted separately, allowing each individual to speak from their own experiences and perspective. The goal is not only to understand how the family members and others around the person view her or him but also how they view each other and the relationships in the web of life around the person that existed prior to and during the person's psychosis. In hearing these different perspectives, the counselors and peer specialists should seek to avoid seeing one or another's perspective as more important or accurate than others but rather as competing perspectives and voices within the person in psychosis. It is also helpful to think of oneself as a detective seeking to put together a picture of the person that includes not only his or her persona, shadow, traumas, issues and relationships but also those of the people in the web of life around her or him.

While preparing for a long-term process, initial assessments should also be looking for the possibility that short term treatments may be possible. In the case of psychosis brought on by excited states, such as G-10, resolving the initial crisis may be as easy as helping the person to get needed sleep and then enter into a program that reorients the person to reality and applies their relevant insights to their life. In situations like those of Ron Coleman and Eleanor Longden, the individuals had strong insight into their experiences as being personal ones, were willing to cooperate with treatment and could have been given tools to help them with the recovery process. Instead, all of these individuals were subjected to needless forced treatments and medication, substantially worsening their lives and providing little if any benefit to their initial problems.

In asking questions about the person's life content, it is important ask the people being interviewed specific questions that allow them to convey their unique individual perspectives. In addition to the more obvious questions that are asked about people's lives, it is important to ask the following questions.

- "What do you want to tell me about the person?"
- "What do you want to tell me about his/her family?"
- "What are the important qualities of person?"
- "What are important qualities of her/his family?"
- "What are important qualities of the person's present and any previous communities?"
- "What has the relationship(s) between the person and his or her present and any previous community been like?
- "What are things and issues that the person cares a lot about?"
- "When were times of stress for the person?"
- "What was the source of the stress for the person and how did he/she react?"
- "When were times of stress for her/his parents?"
- "What was the source of stress for the parents and how did they react?"
- "What were times of stress for the person's siblings?"
- "What was the source of stress for the siblings and how did they react?"

- "What has your relationship with the person been like over the years you've known him/her?"
- "What are other people's relationships with the person like?"
- "Who does the person confide in?"
- "Who does the person trust the most?"
- "What are your ideas about the connection between all these aspects of the person's life and the person's beliefs and experiences during psychosis and in the months and possibly years prior to its onset?"

It is noteworthy that through the process of asking these same questions of people over years of practice, professionals will begin to see patterns between the relationships people have with their parents, siblings, friends and community and the content of their psychosis. In doing so, the understanding of psychosis and how to respond to it will be greatly aided.

As these interviews are being conducted, there are a number of steps that can be taken to help prepare both the person and the people around him or her for the next steps. Family members, friends, and clinicians involved may want to read *Schizophrenia: A Blueprint for Recovery's* first chapter and Appendices A, B, C and E to understand the experiences of people in psychosis. As indicated before, if possible the environment around the person in psychosis should be arranged to maintain peacefulness and positivity, following the description in the handbook's second chapter. The treatment team should also review the handbook's Chapter Two material on the Mentor/Realist Team approach. Based on the circumstances and personalities involved, individuals choose someone to have the mentor relationship with the person. In some cases, the person in psychosis will make a connection with someone on the treatment team or among his or her family and friends and a natural affinity will begin that makes it clear that the person in psychosis is "choosing" a mentor.

As a dialogue begins, the counselor or peer specialist, acting as the mentor, gives a copy of the Appendix E essay, "Saving the World, Saving Yourself" from *Schizophrenia: A Blueprint for Recovery* to the person. When the essay is given, the mentor asks the person to read it and let the mentor know what he or she thinks about the essay.

After the person has read the essay, the mentor and she or he can begin to discuss the person's reaction to the material. After the initial discussion about the material (or at the same time as the essay), the person is given *Working with Voices* by the mentor for the person to use and own as his or her own. *Working with Voices* is a workbook with a step-by-step approach that helps the person experiencing voices and other unusual events to identify the events and their triggers, recognize the emotions connected to the events, seek to identify the sources of the voices, work with the experiences to gain strength in face of them and "give up madness" in favor of the life where the voices, if they continue, are controlled rather than controlling.

The mentor giving the essay and workbook offers, during the first follow-up discussion, to "accompany you on your journey through this material," and share in the person reviewing's unusual experiences, including past experiences. In doing so, the mentor is seeking to create a dialogue with the person and establish a one-on-one counseling relationship aimed at discussing the unusual experiences and beliefs of the person and move the person towards consensus reality.

One issue of concern for people in using *Working with Voices* is the statement early in the workbook that the "voices are real." If the person in psychosis discusses this, the mentor can respond that the voices are really being experienced by the person, but that it is important to understand that these voices and other experiences are not apparently being experienced by others. The mentor should say at this point, "Part of our discussion can be about how you and others see these personal experiences and if and when you feel these personal experiences are helping you get what you want out of life." Since the person's view of his or her experiences may be grandiose, it is important to respect his or her view, recognizing the ways in which the concerns of the person are valid in the larger world, and indicating that the extent of the person's grandiose beliefs being determined to be true will become clear with time. All of this can be used to begin further dialogue and working to help the person gain insight into how outsiders may view their experiences.

It is important for the mentor to convey that what is in the personal experience or personal reality of the person can be very meaningful and important and should be talked about with others. For example, the mentor might move the dialogue with the person towards the belief that it is okay to talk about as these experiences as "real or happening to me but not everyone" and still important, regardless of their overall nature.

As this dialogue continues, the mentor will seek to identify these personal events and beliefs and how this "delusional" content is connected to real life issues and events. To help with this, the mentor will want to ask the person questions during the dialogue, including

- "What is important for me to understand about you?"
- "What is important for me to understand about your experiences?"
- "How does your personal life relate to your experiences?"
- "What do you want to accomplish for yourself through this time?"

An example of the sort of insight that counselors can get through these interviews and dialogues can be exemplified by looking Paris Williams' reporting of the life of "Cheryl" in *Rethinking Madness*. If these questions were initially asked of Cheryl, she would report that, after attending a New Age workshop connecting people to their spirit friends, she came to hear her spirit friends and they are telling her she is a terrible person, the worst soul ever in existence, and God may destroy the world because she is on it.

In looking at this distressing report, it is important to ask, "What are the emotions here and where are they being directed?" The emotions are really extreme anger and hatred directed at Cheryl by these voices, which are largely coming from Cheryl herself. The question becomes, "When was anger and hatred expressed at Cheryl?"

In the interview phase of speaking with family members and friends, the counselors would discover that Cheryl had recently moved to live with a boyfriend and had been rejected by him. Another friend had moved away, causing her to become isolated and feel rejected and alone. In addition to these stresses, she was working with juvenile delinquents who were angry and abusive to her, despite her well-intentioned attempts to help them. Obviously, these voices were probably being triggered in part by Cheryl internalizing her ex-boyfriend's rejection of her, her sense of unworthiness because of a lack of friends and the surrounding voices of the juvenile delinquents she spent the majority of her time with.

As a further note, Cheryl reported to Paris Williams that as a child her parents had been self-involved and that she had a sense of not being loved, though during her psychosis they attempted to express this. Whether this aspect of Cheryl's past is directly or indirectly indicated in the interviews, it is noteworthy that Cheryl's rejection by a boyfriend and isolation is part of a much larger life history and unfolding personal journey in which Cheryl experiences self-loathing that has been internalized from her not experiencing love from others. From these observations, the healing resolution to Cheryl's dilemma becomes clear: finding a way that Cheryl can feel and accept the love of others, especially in her family and her relationships with those close to her. As Paris Williams reports, this gradual transformation in and around Cheryl was the key to her recovery.

Web of life maps

It may be helpful for the counselor or peer specialist to create web of life maps with people, emotions and other things such as alcohol, money and work habits, and draw affinities, parallels and aversions. Making maps that chart the person's psychological and real life movement through these webs of life can be helpful in looking at the underlying events and possible healing resolutions and transformations.

For example, in looking at a young man who has adopted Marxism, despite growing up as a middle-class white person in the United States, one would want to identify the people in his web of life who have money or are very interested in making a lot of money and what his relationships with them are like. In this real life situation, the young man had a father on whom he was economically dependent, despite having argued with the father for years. He also had a career oriented older brother who was rapidly making his way up the corporate ladder while he spiraled into deeper and deeper dysfunction. In time, the young man would reveal that the older brother had severely abused him when they had been growing up and this abuse was one of the causes of his own dysfunction. In mapping out these relationships in this web of life, the anger and abuse aimed at the young man by wealthy and money-oriented men in his family had been associated with their focus on material gain and was being reacted to by adopting a philosophy where those with money are the enemy. It is significant that this sort of personal world analysis of preferences for outer-world philosophies and religions is frequently useful, regardless of one's view of the validity or non-validity of the philosophy.

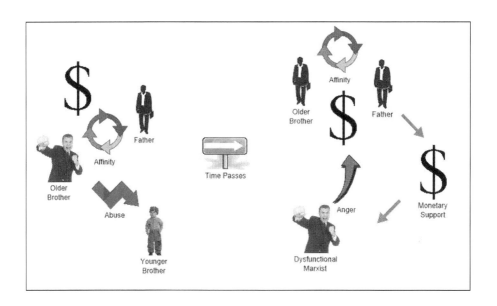

Changes in one's web of life map as time and events go by are also very important. Looking at changes in the person and his or her web of life over time has parallels to Narrative therapy and may be thought as similar to creating story boards for movies, in which the main events of the plot are drawn to highlight the key factors in both the environment and how these factors affect the person's journey.

In the case of Haley, it is helpful to construct three maps, one prior to her religious conversion, one during her time with the conservative church and one after her Mom's death. In the first map, Haley is still connected to her family, repeating and extending her mother's addictions and anger by strong addictions to alcohol and street drugs and a cynical rage expressed through Satanism. In this map, despite the anger between her and her Mom, there is a strong affinity in terms of the sort of life that both generations of the family have and a parallel direction of self-destruction by both the mother and the daughter.

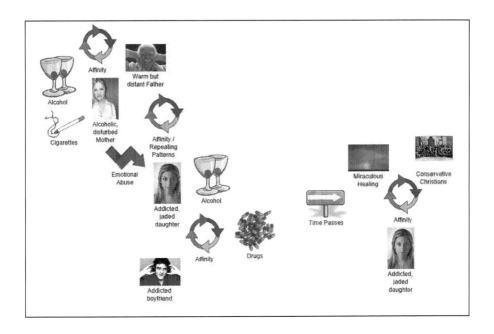

In the map after Haley's miraculous religious conversion, Haley has reacted to her repeating of family patterns by escaping addiction into a religious group that strengthens her desire to remain abstinent and expressed her anger at her family by claiming that they are held in harsh judgment by her god. In this map, the family and she no longer share affinity. In place of that, Haley has affinity with people who claim to be the polar opposite of her earlier life and her family's culture, creating a huge divide between Haley, her family and her old web of life. However, it is important to note that, despite the veneer of judgment and being a zealot, Haley has both deep fears that she will be judged harshly by her god and wishes for her addicted, self-destructive mother the same miraculous liberation that Haley received when she accepted Jesus.

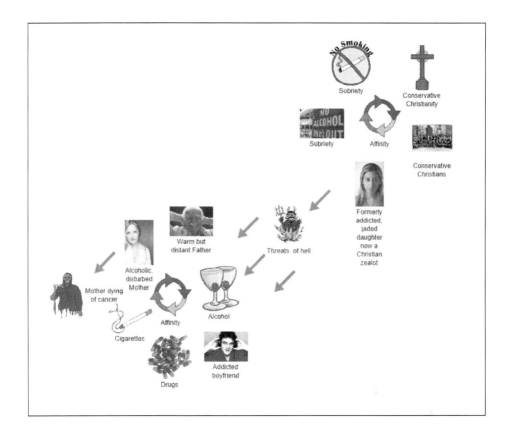

It is significant that in this web of life, especially as Haley's terminally ill mother declines while refusing to give up alcohol and cigarettes, there is no middle ground for Haley to turn to. The people in her web of life are either irreverent addicts and enablers or harshly judgmental religious conservatives who condemn most of humanity as hellbound. Had there been a third part of the web which would push for sobriety but also for moderation and acceptance of Haley's parents as flawed but not condemned people, Haley would have had a true sanctuary to turn to after the death of her Mom.

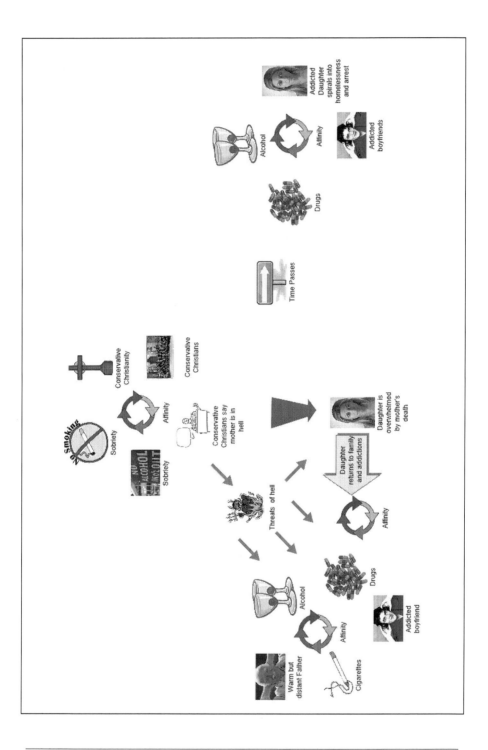

In looking at Haley's web of life map after her Mom has passed, it becomes clear that Haley's love of her Mom has created a crisis of faith that has left Haley alone in the world. At this point, Haley is left with the choice of either believing that her mother has been condemned by her god or that her religion, the source of her strength keeping her own addictions at bay, is false. As a measure of Haley's love of her mother and the real quality of her character, she rejects her church, unable to bear their condemnation of her troubled mother. In this web of life map, her family has largely disintegrated; she has separated from her church and no longer has affinity with them. Without a strong support group to catch her, she falls back into addiction almost as if wishing to follow her mother's fate out of Haley's love for her. As a result of her web of life not having someone to act as a middle ground to keep her sober yet not unfairly condemn her family, Haley spirals into a grief-fueled addiction and is arrested. Ironically, through this arrest she is finally given the middle-ground support she needs to lead a sober, pious but nonjudgmental life.

In looking at a similar set of maps for Mike, the direction of both his psychosis and his life becomes clear. In the pre-psychosis map, Mike is having conflict with both his original family and with his wife, but according to Mike's later insights, the relationship between his father and mother and between him and his wife is very similar. Like other young people, including Haley, Mike was repeating negative patterns from his original family, creating an affinity between his family and himself, despite the conflict between them. His pacifism and other ideals, developed during his teenage years, can be represented as a thought balloon that is disharmonious with his real life.

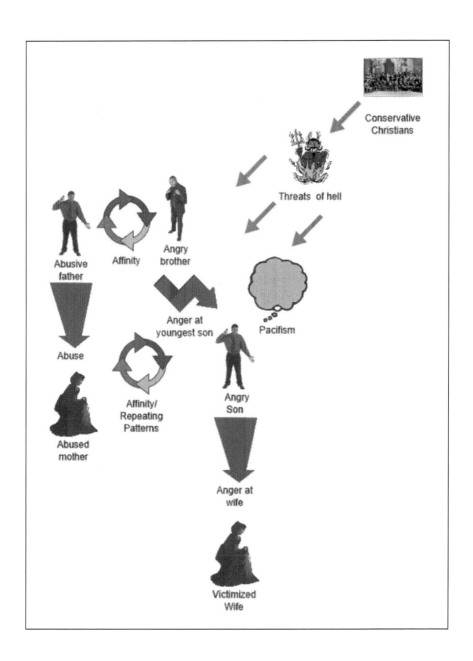

At this stage, he is unconscious of the family and personal factors that have resulted in his severely troubled marriage, as well as being unconscious of the effect that being molested by a brother was having on his life. The map is notable for both its conflict in almost all of the significant relationships around Mike and, ironically, the affinity of the relationships despite this conflict. Surrounding this troubled family is a judgmental, conservative religious community that is condemning all involved. It is an explosive web of life moving towards critical mass.

In the map of Mike's web of life during psychosis, the same conflict exists externally but there are new elements. In a desperate attempt to maintain stability during the onset of his psychosis, Mike has reached out to a feminist woman and her friends. Remarkably, the woman and her friends have responded with concern and support. This new element in the web of life represents a reaction-formation to both Mike's family and community up until now and a continuation of his reaction against the conflict around him that was first expressed by his ideals of pacifism and, now, by feminism. In this phase, Mike is fully psychotic yet becoming aware of the factors that have resulted in his anger and the conflict in his original and chosen families. With this web of life, his affinity is now more in relationship to this new group of people even as he remains in conflict with his family members. A thought balloon representing Mike's emerging ideals of feminism can now be added to the pacifist thought balloon and, unlike the previous web of life map, these ideals have affinity with the group of people around the feminist woman.

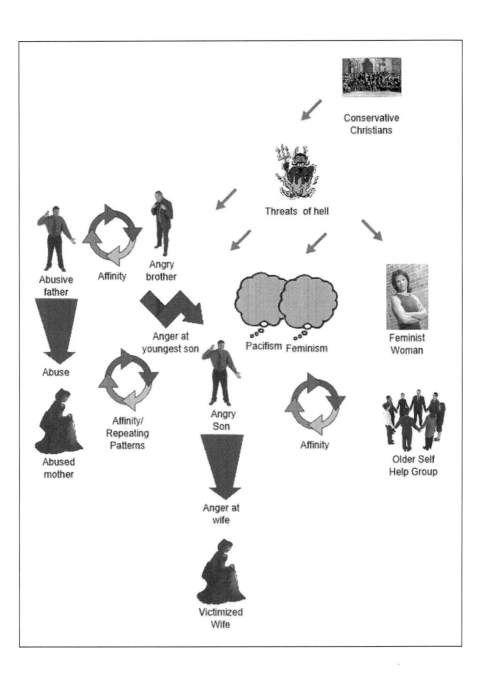

In the post-psychotic web of life, which might be seen as a series of stages evolving towards a new life, Mike's original web of life has been severely disrupted. His marriage is over and his relationships with the men in his family are increasingly distant and lack affinity. Meanwhile, in place of these dysfunctional and conflicting relationships Mike's friendship and affinity with the feminist woman and her friends takes increasingly more importance. During this time, Mike undergoes a series of personal developments that makes his ideals of peacefulness and feminism more and more a part of his real life.

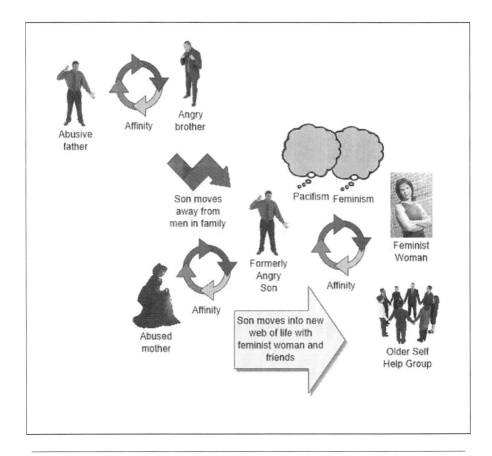

Eventually, Mike's personal development allows him to live his ideals in his personal life. He develops a happy relationship with a woman with affinity with his new personality and in doing so breaks off the unhappy relationships with the men in his family and his old community, completing his reaction-formation from their anger and conflict and from his younger, traumatized self. This transformation, taking over a decade to accomplish, marks positive spiritual and psychological growth that Mike attributes largely to his insights and ideals developed during psychosis.

In comparing the stories of Haley and Mike and the web of life around them, the central difference is that during psychosis Mike had a supportive group of nonjudgmental friends and allies who were able to provide a direction out of his troubled web of life. In the case of Haley, this option was not present in her web of life, giving her no support to allow a complete transformation to occur. This support allowed Mike a much less traumatic journey in the movement towards recovery and transformation compared to Haley.

Beginning transformation, stabilization and recovery

The lesson from the web of life mapping is that a major purpose of care during psychosis is to identify the positive spiritual path that the person is seeking to heal and resolve his or her challenges and for the treatment team to help bring about that crucial web of life support. This support is intended to allow a successful, minimally traumatic conclusion to the spiritual journey of the person. As such, the beliefs and events during psychosis can be seen illustrating the true meaning of the person's life in symbolic terms and to imagine a transformation of these problems. *Crucially, this transformation must not only take place within the mind of the person undergoing psychosis, but also in the web of life she or he is part of.*

To assist in moving the person from psychosis into this transformed self and web of life, the counselor who has given the person the "Saving the World, Saving Yourself" essay and *Working with Voices* should step through this material with the person. The person should be asked to share experiences they have had like the ones described in the material and build up a process by which the experiences become manageable. Care should be taken by the counselor to develop and maintain the trust of the person in psychosis so the person is willing to share her or her journey through this material.

Working with Voices is an invaluable tool in stepping through these experiences, providing direction to help the person identify the triggers for these events, locating the likely sources of these experiences, approaches to manage the events and give up madness. In doing so, the beliefs and experiences that the person undergoing psychosis will be shared with the counselor and allow insight into the relationship between them and the person's life. It is important for person to make these connections for himself or herself, even if therapist may see them clearly.

Working with Voices provides a structure through which the person in psychosis and the counselor take one step at a time towards recovery. The workbook begins by asking the person about goals and fears, has the person describe and analyze their voices and effect they have on him or her, asks about the beginning and the history of the voices, helps identify triggers, connects the person to support from others and "trialogue" with the voices for help, has the person identify coping strategies, begins the person on review of her or his life history to analyze the relationship between real events and the voices. The workbook also includes the possibility of using medication and encourages the person to give up madness.

As this process unfolds, the counselor should try to see how the person's beliefs and experiences are trying to elevate the person's life and pursue a healing resolution. This resolution, which is the key to the transformation being sought, may at first be envisioned in highly symbolic and universal ideals and beliefs. Moving these ideals into concrete form in the person's web of life is essential for the successful conclusion of their spiritual journey.

The Open Dialogue technique of developing a shared vocabulary that is used to describe events should be practiced with the person. Different people express their experiences differently and coming to agreed-on words that express the events allows for terminology that can be used to discuss the events and seek resolution. The counselor and treatment team should seek to convey range of interpretations for events, such as comparing and contrasting different interpretations for hallucinations, visions and voices and delineating the differences between symbolically meaningful events and ideas and random "static" and delusions that result from jumping to conclusions and misperceptions. The expressed and real purpose of this will be to focus the person on "getting what you want out of life—being happy and having your life work – by working through and giving up madness."

In addition to this, a best practice approach would seek to set up a Hearing Voices Group of people who are experiencing voices and hallucinations to serve as group counseling. This group should follow the form and approach advocated by Ron Coleman, in line with the workbook that the person is given. Depending on treatment team, another person can act as a Consensus Realist as described in the second chapter of *Schizophrenia: A Blueprint for Recovery.*

As this process continues, the staff should help the person implement Personal Medicine habits by adding to treatment plan and regular interview questions, such as "What helps you when you are blue?", "What do you enjoy doing?", "What makes your life meaningful?", "What are activities that relieve stress?" and so forth. As the person gives answers to these questions, effort should be made to make sure the person can begin to do these positive, enriching activities in his or her daily life. This approach is contained within the CommonGround software package developed by Pat Deegan. If the questions are used outside that package, the staff should work with Pat Deegan's organization to ensure these are carried out correctly.

In general, the relationship between the counselor and the treatment team and the person in psychosis should follow the outline of the relationships of the Understanding Mentor and Consensus Realist in the second chapter of *Schizophrenia: A Blueprint for Recovery.* While these relationship modes may come naturally for some people, training for these relationship approaches is not presently available for those who would like it. Fortunately, this approach is similar enough to the LEAP model that attending LEAP training will suffice provided that the process of LEAP is applied to the transformation rather than simply to medication compliance. This training is available through the LEAP Institute.

It is important to recognize that the LEAP approach itself does not have insight into some of the more important aspects of psychosis and is primarily concerned with medication compliance. Accordingly, the training should be seen within the overall approach of the Combined Toolkit. The counselor and others should seek to use the LEAP elements of Understanding Listening and empathy to find agreement on positive and consensus reality beliefs, and use the Cognitive Behavioral Therapy element to lessen self and other harmful beliefs.

This model can also be used to discuss the possibility of medication to stem unwanted events, but such discussions should not be the most central part of the combined toolkit. Discussion by the Understanding Mentor of using medication should be delayed until a sense of trust and understanding can be established between the Understanding Mentor and the person undergoing psychosis, following the stages of this of relationship outlined in the second chapter of *Schizophrenia: A Blueprint for Recovery*. This approach is akin the optimal use of medication advocated by some.

Insofar as the use of medication goes, there are four stages to the process:

1. Prior to trying medication, dialogue with the person is established to calm him or her and facilitate the recognition that the experiences of psychosis are personal ones that are not shared by others.

2. If hallucinations and other events are not diminished or eliminated by this point the person is encouraged to suggest and try solutions to reduce and control the events, provided the solutions do not risk the wellbeing of the person or others.

3. Should these attempts fail, the individual is encouraged to try medication to stem the symptoms.

4. If the symptoms are not stopped by medication use or the person prefers other methods to manage the symptoms, alternative approaches are used to maintain stability.

This approach, which can cycle back to #2 if not effective, is similar to the later stages of the relationship with the Understanding Mentor discussed in the second chapter of *Schizophrenia: A Blueprint for Recovery*.

Moving into stability and post-psychosis

As the person moves towards increasing stability and a calmer, happier life, the treatment team creates a WRAP plan with the person to maintain and increase stability. With the already introduced Personal Medicine practices and other habits developed in the psychotic stage, a staff member—ideally a peer specialist—trained in WRAP works out a WRAP plan with the person. This WRAP plan will flesh out the Personal Medicine approach to cover all aspects of stability, ranging from habits during positive times to fall back plans and trusted others to turn to during stress, turmoil and crises.

The reality checking rules outlined in the third chapter of *Schizophrenia: A Blueprint for Recovery* should be introduced to the person and habits that follow the rules in some form should be encouraged and implemented. These reality checking rules will help the person determine personal from consensus experiences and allow them to become aware at an early stage when they are having a return to symptoms.

As the state of psychosis is resolved the "Counseling for Self Understanding" chapter in *Schizophrenia: A Blueprint for Recovery* should be followed to complete the person's long-term transformation as well as aid her or his recovery. Some of the earlier stages should have already occurred, at least in part, during the reading of *Working with Voices*. These include grounding the person in daily life, sorting out personal from consensus events and events that are meaningful from events that random or meaningless and connecting the person's life to events during psychosis.

In addition to these stages discussed in the handbook, the person will be encouraged to identify people in his or her face-to-face web of life to check reality with person. These individuals will be trustworthy and willing to help the person identify when events are shared and when they are occurring just for the person. Ideally, the person should identify someone to do this in each physical location that the person frequents in her or his daily life.

With psychosis either overcome, or with symptoms that are increasingly manageable and reality checking in place, the person is ready for a long-term evaluation of her or his experiences through following the remaining stages of the post-psychotic counseling process. Because of the emotionally powerful and stressful nature of the process, it is essential that the person have a stable and manageable life to maintain their strength during this time.

As the person's counseling continues, he or she will begin to reveal secrets and traumas. Encouraging these shadow elements to be discussed and helping the person get a picture of her or her life with these elements conscious is necessary to complete the counseling. Ideally, the person will be able to outline a personal biography that includes these difficult aspects of their life.

At the same time, the person's secrets will point to the need to face and resolve character flaws. It is helpful for the person to have the treatment team connect the traumas that occurred prior to the flaws taking form so that the person is able to withstand the harsh self-criticism that often accompanies facing character flaws. Other aspects which play into the development of character flaws, such as poor guidance and neglect by significant others and people in authority, are important to bring into the discussion of character flaws.

Combining these various shadow elements allows the person to have an autobiographical outline that she or he will be able to use to review the events of psychosis and draw connections between the meaningful, symbolic beliefs and the real events of his or her life. In doing so, determining the lessons to be learned and identifying real solutions to move toward are central to completing the journey of psychosis.

As indicated in *Schizophrenia: A Blueprint for Recovery*, it is not uncommon for mentally ill people to undergo religious conversions during and after psychosis. Like the experiences of Haley, these religious conversions can have very positive effects, despite the rigidity and harsh judgments that can accompany them. Integrating these personal religious conversions as part of the ongoing resolution, both encouraging the person to modify her or his rigidity while having the treatment team and those in the web of life around the person recognize the positive aspects of the conversion are important in balancing the counseling process with the emerging identity of the person.

Moving the person toward attaining inner peace is a central goal of maintaining stability. Both seeking to have internal contradictions and conflict resolved and developing habits of relaxation, introspection and stress release are ways to cement a new way of life that allows for increased adaptability and a day-to-day calmness and stability. Likewise, using approaches that help resolve trauma is essential to allowing the person an inner peace that eluded him or her before.

As the implementing of resolutions to the shadow problems of trauma, previously undisclosed secrets, and character flaws is carried out, the person will be developing a new identity that is a transformed version of her or his earlier self. This transformation will necessarily have to occur on a concrete level in the daily life of the person in the web of life around him or her. As such, it can represent challenges for others who may not want the transformation to occur because the changes it implies for them. Seeking an Open Dialogue-like approach to group counseling with those around the person may be necessary to prevent a sudden and dramatic conflict between the person and those who resist the changes she or he are making. In some cases, the person may have no alternative but to leave her or his former web of life so that the person's new identity can take hold in a more harmonious and welcoming environment.

Despite the concerns and biases in most secular counseling, having the person review the mystical implications of their experiences is often a deeply rewarding phase of the review of psychosis. Being able gain a sense of spirituality and faith through this review is a way to balance the secular and practical concerns of surviving psychosis with the promise of the experience to provide spiritual insights. It can be helpful to have the person identify ways to maintain an introspective spirituality—such as keeping a dream journal, observing coincidences and synchronicities, and studying ways to enhance intuition—can help satisfy any desire the person has to make spirituality part of their daily life.

In addition to these stages, identifying people in the person's web of life who are committed to helping the person implement a healing resolution in the long term is very helpful in aiding complete transformation. This can range from self-help groups, members of counseling groups, members of the person's spiritual group, friends or even life partners. If these individuals are not present in the person's life, having her or him clearly identify what these people will be like and what he or she will want to complete the transformation that attains her or his spiritual goals. Identifying such people is essential because, in cases of personal transformation, just as in cases of overcoming addictions, changes in the web of life around the person are crucial to lasting and complete spiritual growth.

ADDITIONAL ASPECTS OF CARE

Building working relationships

Despite the widespread belief that there are no real means to communicate and work with someone in psychosis, there are actually a number of different approaches available that allow people to build relationships. Central to all approaches is that a relationship of trust is established between the person in psychosis and those around him or her. The relationship of trust is essential to gaining the confidence of the person and working with him or her to resolve the problems of her or his life.

In *Schizophrenia: A Blueprint for Recovery*, a team approach is described which has different people playing different roles with the person. The "Understanding Mentor" builds trust with the person, becomes a confidant and works on finding solutions to the person's problems. The "Consensus Realist" focuses discussion on practical problems the person faces and having the person getting his or her life to work so she or he can have what is wanted in life. The two relationships work together to jostle the person's mind to think about his or her life in alternative and meaningful ways and finding solutions that resolve not only the psychosis but also other issues.

In Cognitive Behavioral Therapy (CBT), a counselor encourages the discussion of the person's beliefs and experiences. While listening attentively, the counselor also provides alternative, calming explanations for the delusional beliefs and hallucinatory events that the person relates. With the goal of "normalizing" the person's beliefs, the counselor works as a sounding board that gives the person more common viewpoints for her or his experiences. CBT is also used to teach the person to do CBT on his or her own so that once the counseling ends the person has greater ability to avoid and overcome the leaps in faith and jumping to conclusions that mark the psychotic mindset.

The approach of Listen-Empathize-Agree-Partner (LEAP) uses both Understanding Listening from Rogerian therapy and CBT to create a relationship of trust between the person in psychosis and others and to dialogue about her or his experiences. This approach is used primarily to gain the person's compliance with medication and can be effective in doing so. It has commonality with the team approach of the "Understanding Mentor/Consensus Realist" and has the benefit of being more structured, able to be used by a single caretaker and having training available for its practice. However, for the purpose of the toolkit it is best seen as the start of a much deeper relationship than simple medication compliance. LEAP and the other relationship models listed here can be used as the foundation for separating out meaningless from meaningful content and partnering to help bring about a transformation in the person's life.

The Open Dialogue approach to counseling is another way to establish a relationship of trust with the person and to maintain a dialogue that brings the person's experiences and beliefs into the realm of group consensus. By encouraging an exchange of views and sharing of experiences, the Open Dialogue approach "normalizes" the beliefs of the person in a de facto way within the viewpoints of the significant others—family and friends—around her or him. By maintaining this dialogue, the person is able to better relate the experiences of psychosis to his or her personal world and the common beliefs and experiences shared by people within it.

A fifth approach, Hearing Voices Groups, establishes camaraderie among people in psychosis and works to help the person "gain mastery" over her or his voices and other experiences. This process includes identifying the onset of voices, triggers for the events, positive and negative voices and means to dialogue with and gain control of voices. Through this process, the experience of voice hearing can become a positive means of coping for the person, who comes to use the positive voices to his or her benefit while neutralizing the distressing and negative voices. This approach appears to have the most potential to help people who are resistant to medication, who have side effects from medication or who choose to live a life without medication.

All of these approaches to developing relationships with the person in psychosis have merit in different situations. In the cases of CBT and LEAP, training is readily available in the United States. The similarities of LEAP to the Understanding Mentor approach allow the LEAP training to be substituted for it. This training can then be used in conjunction with the material in *Schizophrenia: A Blueprint for Recovery* to expand past the limits of the LEAP view of psychosis. While Open Dialogue and Hearing Voices Groups are very limited within the United States, advocates of these approaches are working diligently to expand their availability.

Improving self-care

There are several complementary approaches to encouraging people in psychosis and post-psychosis to care for themselves. At the end of the "Saving the World, Saving Yourself" essay, a plan for self-care is mapped out to encourage the person to attend to his or her needs. The self-care is primarily for emotional support and centering, allowing the person to develop daily habits that foster peacefulness, calm and stability. With this approach, the inner calm needed to gain personal strength is advanced.

Personal Medicine, which is part of the CommonGround software by Dr. Pat Deegan, allows the person to identify his or her unique characteristics and desires in regaining a meaningful and enjoyable life. The approach interactively identifies the activities and supports that the person can use to be happy, positive and calm and to take part in meaningful activity. In doing so, the person re-establishes habits that make her or his life uniquely meaningful and enjoyable.

The Wellness Recovery Action Plan (WRAP) developed by Dr. Ellen Copeland can be used to formulate responses for a variety of events and stress levels. By creating individualized plans, the person's WRAP can create positive life habits and prepare for stressful events and crises should they arise As such, WRAP handles the more extreme areas of concern that might interfere with recovery. All three of these approaches are available within the United States, and can be used in any combination to work with the specific needs of the person.

Approaches to healing trauma

Trauma is a significant factor in many people's lives. Resolving trauma for people who experience psychosis is essential to recovery and transformation. Fortunately, there are different approaches that are useful for healing trauma. Eye Movement Desensitization and Reprocessing (EMDR) Therapy has a substantial history indicating success in healing the effects of trauma. Using approaches aimed at reprocessing traumatic events within the brain of the person, EMDR can relieve anxiety and resolve flashbacks of pain and anger that arise from recalling traumatic events. Like EMDR, CBT can also be used to help resolve trauma.

Re-Evaluation Counseling (RC), which is one kind of self-help group, also focuses on resolving trauma and the habits that have formed out of trauma. RC works by encouraging people to fully experience the traumatic events at a deeply emotional level and thereby "cleans up the incident," relieving the person of the painful experience and the negative patterns associated with it. It is important to note that many RC self-help groups are strongly against the use of medication and therefore are more helpful for those who view themselves as survivors of the mental health system rather than those who are on medication and who are successful in being able to manage their lives. Also, like all self-help and professional counseling groups, the effectiveness of RC can depend on the personalities and skills of the people delivering the counseling. Those working with RC groups should have relationships of trust with people outside the group to serve as sounding boards for the counseling.

The focus on emotions in Re-Evaluation Counseling has many parallels with Processed Experiential or Emotion Focused therapy, which seeks to increase awareness of the emotions that underlie everyday conversation and events. Emotion Focused therapy can be used in parallel with RC and may also be useful for doing the sort of analysis that began the first passage's examination of the personal world.

Emotional Connecting, emPowering and Revitalizing (eCPR) is a recently formulated approach developed by peers to help people overcome trauma and revitalize their lives. Seeking to provide a generic cognitive approach to resolving trauma through developing connection with the person and identifying means for him or her to regain control of their lives, eCPR may be used to encourage the person to re-engage in his or her life. While estimating the effectiveness of this new approach is difficult at this time, eCPR may prove to be another useful tool in helping people overcome trauma.

Psychological trauma involves not only healing past emotional wounds but also identifying a way to avoid future trauma. Many people live in relationships with past trauma embedded in them, especially in the case of abuse in the family or face-to-face community. Susan Forward's acclaimed work, *Toxic Parents*, as well as many other books, outlines approaches to both heal trauma and deal effectively with family or community members who are abusive or calloused to past abuse. While the material in *Toxic Parents* focused on parental relationships, the approach to relationships that she outlines can be used in other relationships, both inside and outside the family. Other books by Susan Forward focus on specific forms of abuse, such as incest, and may prove useful for these specific forms.

The role of trauma in triggering hallucinations and delusions is also significant. Like the intrusive symptoms of PTSD and reoccurring patterns discussed in RC, when events around a person in psychosis touch on past trauma, hallucinations and/or delusions are often triggered. By reducing the impact of trauma on people like me who are prone to psychosis, the impact of intrusive symptoms ranging from powerful emotions to hallucinations to uncontrolled behavioral patterns is reduced.

Resources for the family

There are various resources available for families to help deal with loved ones in crisis as well as their own needs. The National Alliance on Mental Illness (NAMI) is the most commonly recognized advocacy group and has long-established courses and support groups such as "Family-to-Family" which are aimed at educating families about mental illness. NAMI was primarily created and until recently made up of family members. To a large degree, NAMI is a resource more for family members than for people with mental illness. In the various debates on treatment options, until recently NAMI has been a more conservative member of the debate. As such, NAMI is suited for helping family members maintain strength during the hard times of family members' illnesses. The Depression-Bipolar Support Alliance (DBSA) is a similar organization focusing on families and people with depression and bipolar symptoms.

A recently formed organization, Mother Bear – Families for Mental Health, has a philosophy that is much less oriented toward the medical model than NAMI and is working to establish approaches that are supported by both peer and family organizations. The Mother Bear organization focuses on multiple strategies for recovery, which includes the use of medication when helpful and necessary.

The "Recovering Our Families" online course is an intensive, advanced approach to re-envisioning the person with mental health problems and the family member's relationship to him or her. Done in partnership with Mother Bear, Practice Recovery and Family Outreach and Response the Recovering Our Families course seeks a hopeful, strengths-based approach to families contributing positively to their loved ones' recovery.

Despite the traditional political divides between the traditionally more conservative and family-dominated NAMI organization, and the more progressive and peer-oriented approach of Mother Bear, seeking support from these and other organizations at the same time is recommended. By finding a variety of viewpoints and approaches, families can best be informed about the range of approaches available to helping both themselves and their loved ones.

Advocacy for the person

Jason Lai, a client's rights advocate, compiled a quick and very useful list of qualities of effective advocates for those in need. Family members, friends and professionals can all benefit by following the guidelines below in working on behalf of those in need. Jason kindly agreed to allow me to include these guidelines in this book.

- **Be Organized.** Keep track of whom you have talked to, the agency the person works for, when and where the conversation occurred, what was said and any decisions made. It is helpful to have a notebook/steno pad to keep notes centrally located.

- **Be Articulate.** Seek to be able to share what is going on, what is wrong and what you would like done.

- **Know the system's pressure points/system advocates.** Identify and maintain contact with client rights officers, ombudsmen, your state's Legal Rights Services, your state NAMI and your nearby NAMI and Mother Bear affiliates.

- **Know the appropriate process and follow it.** Ask all of your contacts (caseworkers, counselors, advocates, fellow family members, others) on how the system is supposed to work; follow the process and document that you are doing that; if procedures are not being followed correctly, "make noise" about these failings in a polite but firm and strong-willed manner.

- **Document and form paper trail.** Save all written correspondences (letters, emails, etc.) and all notes on conversations. Be sure to include dates on all documents.

- **Foster a spirit of collaboration and accountability.** Work to form a team with family members, the person you are advocating for and system staff. Appreciate and validate people when they are helpful or make strides to improve the situation.

Resources for the person

There are numerous resources for the person experiencing psychosis and seeking recovery. Self-help groups and classes, such as NAMI's Person to Person, Schizophrenics Anonymous, Hearing Voices Groups, and the Recovering Our Families course are all groups that can help the person deal with their experiences. The more traditional and conservative approaches such as the Person to Person course may appeal to some, while spiritually inclined people may be helped with Schizophrenics Anonymous. For those seeking a more progressive approach, the Hearing Voices Groups, where available, can help in creating a fellowship of people experiencing similar symptoms while Recovering Our Families can work to resolve communication and relationship problems within families.

In the last two decades peer organizations have been developed, often supported by state mental health funds, helping to support peer specialists and provide some advocacy for peers separate from families. Networking with these peer organizations is possible through the National Empowerment Coalition website.[5] In doing so both people in psychosis and various stages of recovery can move from receiving support to potentially becoming peer specialists and benefitting others. Unfortunately, since these organi-

---

[5] http://www.power2u.org/

zations are largely reliant on state funding, their ability to serve others is largely dependent on the attitudes of mainstream funders who may have little knowledge of effective mental health treatments.

In terms of creating positive atmospheres and treatments for people in psychosis, residential communities such as CooperRiis Healing Community are models for what could be the standards of treatment for mental illness. Unfortunately, the costs of residential communities such as these can be prohibitive. Even so, looking to these communities as centers creating new and effective means to help people in need can be helpful in transferring their approaches to a local setting.

OTHER TOOLS

It is important to acknowledge that there are numerous other resources and approaches that are not discussed here. These approaches range from Clubhouses and various day treatment programs to Windhorse to Soteria house to Cognitive Enhancement Therapy, to less-structured Hearing Voices groups, to a wide variety of other approaches and tools. The fact that these other resources and approaches are not discussed here is not because I do not believe they are effective, but because I have limited knowledge of their results. This is my failing, not theirs.

It is important to note that additional approaches and tools are being created regularly as the process of lived experience and giving back in response to having received support is ongoing. Any complete review of approaches to working with schizophrenia would be both lengthy and soon out-of-date as new approaches are created.

The tools in this toolkit are a starting point for inquiry. A person might, for example, use this protocol for a year or two, and then begin to tweak it, adding additional approaches or modifying it by adding components for substance abuse or other issues. Ideally, the reader will see this material as a means to discover, through your own experience and native genius, the most effective approaches for the many different forms of "psychosis" we have been taught to lump together as one condition. Hopefully, professionals will be comfortable using different tools to fit the unique circumstances of the person's life. These will undoubtedly include tools not discussed here, some of which have yet to be formulated.

COUNSELING AND ISSUES WITH COUNSELORS

The toolkit that is outlined here is marked by substantial amounts of counseling, both from professional counselors and from self-help groups. While the toolkit advocates counseling, it is important to note that any counseling is only as effective as the counselor who carries it out. Counselors who attempt to implement the toolkit should work with special focus on gently allowing the person in psychosis and post-psychosis to chart his or her own course to recovery and transformation rather than impose the counselor's values and ambitions onto her or him. Likewise, the theoretical perspectives of the counselor should be seen as pointers to possible insights rather than laws of human behavior. Just as individual people from the same family and circumstance vary enormously in our personalities, emotions and ambitions, people from different backgrounds vary enormously in what they want out of life and in which web of life they will thrive. Solutions for each person should be made to fit the individual with as much input from the person who is undergoing the transformation as possible.

As someone who has been through decades of both self-help and professional counseling, I have benefitted enormously in hearing the perspective of others. In many cases, these perspectives have been supportive, however in both self-help groups and professional counseling the tendency for the person playing the counseling role to project their experiences and preferences has been a consistent challenge for me to recognize and overcome. At this point I am quietly amused when a professional counselor chooses to "challenge" my statements about my beliefs and experiences. I have enough sounding boards in real life that support my eccentric but personally meaningful view of reality that I am not damaged by being challenged by someone I see once a month or less. I am amused because invariably in my experience, when professional or self-help counselors and I have conflicted on the best course for me, it has been because the best course for me has been one that would not be acceptable to the counselor in his or her individual circumstances. "This would be a terrible idea for me," the counselor seems to think, "So I have to convince poor Milton that it is a terrible idea for him." As I say, I appreciate the humor in the situation.

Overall the counseling and spiritual choices I have made have served me well, but the same counselors and the same spirituality would not benefit others nearly as well. For those who wish to counsel people using this toolkit there needs to be a constant taking of the perspective of the other person. A counselor may have, for example, been terribly abused by a father and helped by a mother, but the person being counseled might have the reverse situation and have a path for his or her personal transformation that is difficult, even repugnant, to the inner feelings of the counselor. In these situations, whether the counselor is a professional or part of a self-help group, consciously reviewing the similarities and differences in each person's life is essential in preventing the counselor from projecting our personal journey onto those we are trying to help.

APPROACHES OTHER THAN THE TOOLKIT

The toolkit outlines various approaches and is centered on an intensive counseling aimed at both introspection and transformation. For some people, such work is either extremely painful emotionally or simply unnecessary, making large portions of the toolkit counterproductive. This is an important recognition, especially because attempting to force introspective counseling onto someone prior to the person being ready—if they ever will be—can be damaging to recovery. Some people do not feel comfortable facing their inner self for no other reason than they find introspection unpleasant, painful and unnecessary. For these individuals, the central parts of the toolkit will not work.

In looking at these circumstances, it is important to note that some people who still experience symptoms are functional through using a number of distraction and withdraw approaches. By looking at the lives and approaches of remarkably successful people who live with symptoms we can see other approaches. Recovery pathways that are modeled on Keris Myrick's approach[6] may also be developed or may emerge from the studies of Elyn Saks[7] on coping strategies of high-functioning people with schizophrenia. In circumstances where the introspection of the toolkit is not desired or is counterproductive, these pathways may provide solutions that cannot be attained elsewhere.

NON-MEDICAL APPROACHES

In addition to the medically-oriented approaches discussed above, numerous non-medical approaches can be very effective in helping both recovery and spiritual growth. Eastern disciplines including various forms of meditation, yoga, Tai Chi, and other practices are valuable tools for deepening one's connection to the spirit and to gaining insight, control and compassion within one's mind.

Guided meditations and creative visualizations can also be used to foster a positive and stronger inner self. Likewise, studying dreams can be helpful in identifying one's inner emotional terrain and observing inner changes over time. It should be noted that guided meditations should be primarily used at this stage for relaxation and self and other affirming creative visualizations.

More extensive and complex forms of spiritual exploration such as shamanic journeying and meditative vision questing—as well as actual vision questing—are enormously complex and sometimes highly difficult and potentially

---

[6] http://www.nytimes.com/2011/10/23/health/23lives.html

[7] http://weblaw.usc.edu/centers/saks/

damaging approaches to intensive spiritual experiences. Anyone who is interested in these advanced approaches should have moved well past the early recovery stage and have identified a respected and experienced guide to help move into this complex and deeply powerful aspect of spirituality.

Nutritional support for oneself, both for overall health and for the nervous system, is also a very useful approach. *Prescription for Nutritional Healing*, a thorough resource book for a large variety of ailments with support and healing through vitamins and supplements, is an essential guide for healthy recovery and maintenance. Its value in maintaining health cannot be understated.

Finally, in future years, seeking input from Indigenous cultures with knowledge of vision quests seems to me a reasonable recognition of how much Western culture simply does not know about the realm of psychosis. The possibility of much greater insight, in terms of symbols, in healing and in applying the knowledge learned from our journeys through psychosis can best be sought through Indigenous cultures that have millennia of experience with using these experiences to benefit themselves and the individuals who are prone to having vision quests.

WITNESSING THE SPIRITUAL JOURNEYS OF PEOPLE SHARING A WEB OF LIFE

Psychosis is frequently a spiritual journey by a person in response to his or her web of life. In this journey we seek a transformation of both who we are and the environment in which we live. The professionals involved hopefully will be able to witness a spiritual journey not only of the person but everyone in the person's web of life as they interact, change and grow (or refuse to grow) in response to each other.

The medical model is most effective in treating people like me who require medication, do well on medication and do not suffer severe side effects. When those who do not need medication are subtracted from the total percentage that E. Fuller Torrey indicates benefit from medication, those like me may be as high as 50% of those who suffer psychosis. In its expressed purpose of stopping the events of psychosis, this means that the medical model only effectively serves one out of two people, which is a disturbing deviation from the accepted beliefs for the past four decades. It is important for me to acknowledge that the medical model has benefitted me personally; it is also important for me to acknowledge that it has caused unnecessary suffering to many.

In looking at the critiques of the medical model that are supplied by some peer leaders, on the other hand, what is lacking is a comprehensive approach to working with people in psychosis without reliance on medication. Without a comprehensive approach, the reforms being advocated by progressives in the medication debate fail to supply alternatives that are readily available to those in the United States. The combined toolkit in this book is a first attempt to provide an alternative. Readers are encouraged to test and revise it as needed or to provide alternatives that realistically face the challenge the life-threatening condition of untreated psychosis. Resolving this challenge allows psychosis to not only be endured but also become the foundation for life-changing psychological and spiritual growth.

For me, the area where the medical model misses the greatest possible chance for healing is in creating the often inaccurate belief that the symbolic content of psychosis is not relevant to people's lives—and not simply the lives of people who undergo it, but also for our families, communities, the larger society and, in some ways, the human world as a whole. The events of psychosis occur in the context of the slowly unfolding dramas of our families, communities and larger societal and world issues. While causing misperceptions and exaggerations that bring about a series of crises, in many cases psychosis also allows personal insight and motivation that can transform the person's life.

By creating and maintaining the impression that psychosis is always a random hodgepodge of meaningless delusions, the medical model fails to take advantage of a potent opportunity to help bring about spiritual transformations for people in this challenging and wonderful world. Regardless of whether or not we benefit from the use of medication, as I so fortunately do, the larger questions of our lives are being asked by our journeys through psychosis. By using tools like those outlined in this section, professionals can help people like me with the crucial life transformation we need for a successful conclusion of our lives' spiritual journeys.

APPENDIX A
COMPARISON OF TOOLS IN COMBINED TOOLKIT

CENTRAL ASPECTS OF TOOLKIT

The central aspects of the toolkit are the essay, "Saving the World, Saving Yourself," the mentoring process and the post-psychotic counseling which are outlined in *Schizophrenia: A Blueprint for Recovery* and *Working with Voices*. These central approaches are essentially the pairing of a handbook for those around a person experiencing psychosis and the workbook for those experiencing voices and similar events. There are numerous parallels in the approaches and I see them as differing primarily in the people they are aimed at.

Working with Voices is primarily focused on hearing voices, but this limitation can be overcome by accompanying it with the "Saving the World, Saving Yourself" essay which seeks to describe numerous experiences and beliefs of those who experience psychosis. For those who read the sections of the handbook on the mentoring role and post-psychotic counseling and, at the same time, read the process outlined in *Working with Voices*, the parallel approaches become clear. Some steps in *Working with Voices* are delayed in the *Blueprint* until the post-psychotic counseling phase, but the approach of the workbook can be easily blended with the *Blueprint* on a case-by-case basis.

RELATIONSHIP MODELS

Several models for relationships with people experiencing psychosis are touched on in the toolkit. CBT, LEAP, the Mentor/Realist roles from the *Blueprint*, Hearing Voices groups and Open Dialogue. In terms of availability for training in the United States, only CBT and LEAP are widely available, making their role important for practical purposes if none other.

CBT is an established practice of retraining the person to normalize their thoughts to become more mainstream and less distressing and grandiose. It has a strong track record and decades of practice. Its ability to recognize valid insights and experiences of those in psychosis, however, is dependent on the person practicing CBT. This poses the potential problem that real life issues and insights may be "normalized" out of the person's consciousness, resulting in a poor adaptation and unresolved real life issues.

LEAP is another established practice which incorporates Understanding Listening, empathy and CBT, as well as a means to partner with the person to work together. Training is widely available and its similarity in methodology to the mentor/realist roles in the *Blueprint* allows its training to serve in place of training for mentors and realists. It is also useful in cases where there is a single caregiver or single person in contact with the person in psychosis, whereas the mentor/realist team was developed in situations with multiple people in contact with the person.

The purpose of LEAP is to convince the person to take medication and has little if any insight into the real life elements that are part of psychosis and recovery. As such, it can help resolve some of the symptoms of psychosis while leaving huge areas of a person's life ignored as meaningless delusions. Accordingly, it can actually hinder long term recovery and transformation unless it is paired with the insights into psychosis available through the rest of the toolkit. Seeing LEAP as a segment in the process of the toolkit, rather than as its primary component, is essential for the success of the toolkit.

The Mentor/Realist roles from the *Blueprint* essentially split the Understanding Listening/empathy aspect and the CBT aspect of LEAP into two roles, the mentor and the realist. Developed independently from LEAP, this team approach mimics a common real-life environment for people in psychosis who may be confronted by the medical system and authorities on the one hand (realists) and by well-intentioned friends who are more focused on real life issues that extend past medication (mentors). Potentially a role for peer specialists, mentors can help provide a general sense of the person's thinking and priorities within her or his delusional framework, allowing for teamwork on medical and non-medical issues alike. Being less structured than LEAP and *Working with Voices*, the mentor/realist roles can benefit from combining with these more formalized approaches.

Hearing Voices Groups and Open Dialogue are approaches with track records outside the United States. Hearing Voices Groups, though growing in popularity around the world, have prominent people who are success stories of the approach, including Ron Coleman and Eleanor Longden. I do not know of very much literature which discusses results of Hearing Voices Groups in general and since the purpose of the groups is to teach people how to live with and benefit from the voices, it is difficult to apply measures which are concerned more with stopping these symptoms altogether.

Hearing Voices Groups are themselves very eclectic and my personal recommendation is that groups which have adopted the methodology of *Working with Voices* should be the only ones used. To me, the possibility of groups of people who are hearing voices while using an open-ended structure might meander and fail to support true recovery is high. Hearing Voices Groups are, by their name, primarily focused on people who are hearing voices and may lack the sophistication of more complex hallucinations. Combing these groups with the toolkit outlined in this material, however, will hopefully provide a more robust structure while preserving the self-help approach of the group.

Open Dialogue, which has been practiced for decades in a small community in Northern Finland, has substantial reported rates of success for its area. The approach may be useful in the future for the United States, but actual training is very limited. Open Dialogue is also an intensive counseling approach and getting funding for the approach in the United States will continue to be difficult until mainstream funders begin to refocus treatment on counseling rather than medication.

SELF-CARE

The three forms of self-care mentioned in the toolkit are actually complimentary approaches that cover different but related forms of improving one's life. Personal Medicine is primarily focused on personal maintenance and having a life that is meaningful to the individual person. WRAP aids with personal maintenance but also extends its work to outline approaches to crises. The self-help guidelines that are listed at end of the "Saving the World, Saving Yourself" essay are essentially psychological self-care suggestions focused on maintain inner peace and a positive outlook.

ADOPTING DIFFERENT APPROACHES BASED ON INDIVIDUAL CIRCUMSTANCES

The purpose of the toolkit is to provide a generalized set of treatments that might be used in different combinations with different situations. The table below is meant to be the outline of one partial set of possibilities for treatment that could be used in situations with substantial funding. This example is only intended as one possibility and does not cover all of the treatment tools available in the toolkit.

The purpose of the example is not to outline what a professional should always do in these situations. Instead, it is meant to be a partial example of what a professional might decide to do in these situations. The value of the toolkit is like a real life toolkit for a plumber or an electrician. It is up to the native genius of the people interacting with people in psychosis to use insights provided by first-hand observations to identify the correct tools to use in any given situation.

Example of possible selection of some tools by typology with ideal funding of care.

MEDICATION / PHENOMENOLOGY	SYMPTOMS DIMINISH WITHOUT MEDICATION	SYMPTOMS PERSIST WITHOUT MEDICATION	MEDICATION INEFFECTIVE OR CAUSE SEVERE SIDE EFFECTS
Voices Only	Hearing Voices approach with short-term residential facility	Toolkit protocol with medication and Hearing Voices approach at medium-term residential facility	Hearing Voices approach and Toolkit protocol without medication at medium-term residential facility
Voices and Hallucinations	Hearing Voices approach, short-term residential facility and Toolkit protocol	Toolkit protocol with medication and Hearing Voices approach at medium-term residential facility	Hearing Voices approach and Toolkit protocol without medication at medium-term residential facility
Bipolar Psychosis without voices or hallucinations	Short term residential facility with partial Toolkit protocol*	Toolkit protocol with medication for Bipolar at medium-term residential facility	Toolkit protocol without medication and emphasis on WRAP at medium-term residential facility

*Due to the often short-term nature of bipolar psychosis, it is possible that only the initial phases of the toolkit used to investigate meaning and re-connect the person to consensus thinking would be needed.

RE-CREATING THE PERSON'S WEB OF LIFE

As indicated in the toolkit, the purpose of the toolkit is not to simply suppress symptoms or bring about an internal change within the person, but also to help facilitate a change in the person's surrounding world. Web of life maps can help the treatment team and others see the options the person has or may need to have to accomplish a true healing from the challenges she or he face.

Self-help peer groups, like Hearing Voices Groups and other peer groups can provide the beginning points of changes in the person's web of life. Also, moving through the stages of rejoining the mainstream that is outlined in Chapter Five of the *Blueprint* can help identify new people to share the new identity of the person in post-psychosis. Encouraging the person to volunteer and/or retrain in areas that are concrete expressions of his or her ideals during psychosis can be central to completing transformation.

HEALING TRAUMA

Of the approaches mentioned for healing trauma, EMDR and CBT for trauma are the two best established practices and the ones that I would recommend as a first choice. EMDR has a proven track record and an established structure that makes it effective.

Re-Evaluation Counseling (RC), which is a form of self-help group, seeks to build a non-hierarchal counseling environment and allow the greatest autonomy. There are instances among peers where RC has been effective. However, given the RC view that medication is not a solution in most cases limits the choices that people who experience psychosis can rely on. Likewise, the effectiveness of RC depends on the ability of the members of the group to help each other. Like Hearing Voices Groups without a clear structure, RC may actually interfere with recovery if the group is ineffective.

Emotional Connecting (em)Powering Revitalizing (eCPR) is a new approach that may prove useful for trauma. Training is available and the approach can be implemented in the United States. eCPR, however, has sometimes been advocated as a panacea for all people in all circumstances and I do not see this as a reliable statement. For example, the trauma-focused approach of eCPR could be manipulated by people with personality disorders to focus conversation in self-serving and ineffective means. Likewise, the expectation that eCPR will appeal to the varying personalities of the human world—which ranges from policemen and soldiers on one hand to artists and poets on the other—seems to me to greatly underestimate the role that sensitivity plays in both applying and being helped by a technique like eCPR.

Example of selection of trauma treatment by response to medication.

SYMPTOMS DIMINISH WITHOUT MEDICATION	SYMPTOMS PERSIST WITHOUT MEDICATION	MEDICATION INEFFECTIVE OR CAUSES SEVERE SIDE EFFECTS
EMDR, CBT for trauma, Re-Evaluation Counseling, eCPR	EMDR, CBT for trauma, eCPR	EMDR, CBT for trauma, Re-Evaluation Counseling, eCPR

RESOURCES FOR THE FAMILY AND THE PERSON

As indicated in the toolkit section, there are numerous organizations seeking to aid families and people with mental health challenges, including NAMI and its Family to Family and Person to Person courses, Mother Bear – Families for Mental Health, the Recovering Our Families online course, as well as Schizophrenics Anonymous, peer organizations such as the National Association of Peer Specialists and those listed on the National Empowerment Coalition website, and medium-term residential communities, of which I can personally recommend the CooperRiis Healing Community, are all available for families and people who experience psychosis.

NAMI Family to Family is significantly more influenced by the medical model than the Recovering Our Families online course. While established for much longer than the Recovering Our Families course, the Family to Family course can be argued to be much more dated in terms of its material and to potentially create a situation where the person in psychosis becomes "the identified patient," allowing family members to overlook the family and community patterns which may exacerbate the problems of the person in psychosis.

The Recovering Our Families online course is a very advanced course and for some the material in it is so different from their own thinking and presented in such a rapid manner that keeping up with the curriculum is very challenging. While currently online, the long term plans for the Recovering Our Families course is to create face-to-face groups who will take the course together.

Regardless of possible concerns about these courses, it is very helpful for people to take these courses. Doing so allows people to become aware of many different views and tools in helping with people in psychosis and post-psychosis. It also allows people to meet others who are also dealing with these challenges. In doing so, the ability to get support and knowledge crucial to recovery and transformation is greatly aided.

Peer organizations are opportunities for people who experience mental health challenges to use their lived experiences to benefit each other. Peer organizations often speak of attempting to change the culture around us to follow the more compassionate relationships that peers seek to have with each other. As such, peers are often advocates not simply for each other but for a larger cultural change. Those who advocate for eCPR often see the approach as aimed not simply as resolving trauma but also in making our larger culture more compassionate and humane.

In looking at the many resources for families and people with mental illnesses, it is important to note that when we look at everyday problems—such as work holism, affairs, addictions, racism, single motherhood, physical and emotional abuse, divorce and use of porn—I have seen at least some of these in almost all of the families and communities I have known. While not causing mental illness, these issues along with many other problems of families and communities are wholly relevant to recovery and transformation. Creating treatment approaches that encourage people to face and transcend these problems is crucial to moving our webs of life forward.

While the *Blueprint* discusses resolving character flaws and Ron Coleman's *Recovery: An Alien Concept* discusses taking "ownership" of one's problems, when we examine the resources available for individuals and families it is significant that there are no resources that truly encourage people to face and resolve our moral failures in the style of the twelve steps of Alcoholics Anonymous and Al-Anon. While some may feel that an approach like this invites self-stigma, it is an important part of our spiritual journey to become aware and resolve our character flaws on an ongoing basis.

In working against stigma, it is easy to think of ourselves as victims and to strongly reject any negative stereotypes associated with mental illness. In seeking to focus on our strengths and improve our self-esteem, it is easy to overlook our personal failings. These directions are commonplace for people both inside and outside the mental health community. However, when we overlook our flaws and see ourselves only as victims, spiritual growth is hindered by creating a false self-esteem and a refusal to face and resolve our shortcomings. Having a balanced approach that sees both our strengths and our failings is a central aspect of spiritual growth and transcendence of our life's challenges.

NOTE ON PSYCHOLOGICAL THEORIES

While this book began with touching on a few ideas from Freud and Jung, I personally see different theories as similar to different tools in this toolkit. Theories do not usually apply to everyone or no one; each theory represents part of the human experience. Some theoretical approaches that seem related to the analyses in the first and second passages of this book include Emotion Focused therapy, various psychodynamic theories and Narrative therapy. Looking into these approaches may help understand some people who experience psychosis. While concepts in these theories may not be easily reduced into the concrete indicators needed for "evidence based" support, they allow insight lacking in statistical analyses of the human spirit.

In Paris William's *Rethinking Madness*, numerous theories about the nature of psychosis are reviewed and compared. For further study of theories, *Rethinking Madness* is an excellent beginning. The different theories each have application in varying degrees in different webs of life, where different human cultures hold sway.

An example of this comes from my observation of the use of phallic symbols in the world around me. This tired, old Freudian concept, considered passé in our modern culture, seemed to apply in cases of individuals who I met whose outward persona maintained a rigid disdain for obvious references to sex yet who privately had strong sex drives. One person, a conservative Christian man who was caught printing porn on a company printer, used phallic symbols so blatantly that it was embarrassing to me, though he was unconscious he was using them.

On the other hand, in the humorously bawdy subculture of modern partiers, such phallic references cannot remain unconscious—the fun-loving jokers in the crowd will point them out for a quick laugh, making it impossible for phallic symbols to have secret meaning. As such, even some of the more outdated concepts of Freud may still hold sway in cultures that retain both the public repression of and the secret obsession with sexuality that Victorian "gentlemen" relished. However, this same concept is largely useless in many parts of our society, where sexuality is a conscious and public aspect of life.

Looking at theories as reflecting the author's web of life and having validity in similar webs of life is central to recognizing both the value and limits of all theories. Like Joseph Campbell's analysis of myth which indicated that religious stories are centered in the time and place of the cultures that create them, a theory is most valuable in the web of life that created them and then, to some degree, in webs of life that share characteristics with the original web. Choosing parts of different theories that fit best with the web of life that one is looking at, rather than attempting to make observations conform to a specific theory in its entirety, is central to using theories as additional tools in the toolkit.

APPENDIX B
ADAPTING THE COMBINED TOOLKIT FOR MEDIUM-TERM FACILITIES

The initial presentation of the material in this book was made at the CooperRiis Healing Community in February 2013. As I became familiar with the limited time (six to nine months) that CooperRiis had to work with people in psychosis, I realized that the combined toolkit would take far too long to be used by CooperRiis. Shortly after my visit, I created an outline of a procedure for staff at medium-term residential facilities like CooperRiis to use. The purpose is to begin the steps of the Combined Toolkit and to hand over the care of people who may continue to hallucinate and become delusional after leaving the facility. These beginning steps are aimed at successfully completing at least the five goals below during the stay at the facility.

1. Arrive at point where resident understands that she/he has had and may continue to have non-consensus personal experiences (hallucinations, etc.) and trusts at least one person at the medium-term facility to check reality for him/her and be a sounding board for her/his ideas and beliefs.

2. Have resident identify a person in web of life he/she will be entering who she/he are willing to trust for reality checking and being a sounding

board. Have that person clearly agree to take on this role. Possibilities for this include family, close friends, counselors and clergy.

3. Provide departing resident with the capacity and desire to identify additional people to trust for reality checking and being sounding boards as her/his recovery continues.

4. Identify some of the basic issues of the resident's journey, including triggers, trauma and personal stressors contributing to her/his hallucinations and psychosis and some ways in which the person's spiritual quest symbolizes a creative and positive transformation of those issues.

5. Inform the family and the trusted other(s) of the resident's material in #4 as aspects to consider in the role they will play in the resident's recovery.

To accomplish these goals, the resident is taken through the early steps of toolkit. These early steps include the mentor giving the "Saving the World, Saving Yourself" essay and *Working with Voices* to the person. The counselor will seek to step through the essay and the workbook as far as can be accomplished while accommodating the needs of the person and his or her own absorption of the material. The most important part of this process is to have the person see the value of the process and want to continue it after she or he leave the residential facility. Staff should also interview friends and family members to gather information about the person and what real life events may be contributing to the content of their psychosis.

During the early process of the toolkit protocol, the mentor will seek to normalize resident's perception of visions, voices, etc. as oftentimes hallucinations or "static" which may have no meaning. Events reported by the person from his/her life during the toolkit review are used to accomplish this.

Part of this approach is to define a "vision" as non-consensus personal event that is accurately interpreted for meaning in the person's life and/or prediction of consensus events. On the other hand, hallucinations and static are defined as all other non-consensus events. Keeping in mind that the person may have their own terminology for these two sorts of occurrences and being careful to use agreed-on vocabulary is essential to communication.

Once this agreed view of events is established with the person, the mentor will seek to establish in the resident the need for him or her to have trusted others to help check reality and to be sounding boards to identify non-consensus events. These trusted others, to be chosen by the person, is a way for the person to also identify any meaning that may lie within her or his experiences.

In addition to this work, it is important to

- Establish practices of maintaining inner peace and self-care for the person.
- Identify triggers to help avoid or recognize hallucinations as they occur.
- Identify basic relationships between content of person's life, psychosis and spiritual quest.

- Develop agreed-on approach to minimize non-consensus events.

Accomplishing these goals is central to beginning the person on the toolkit approach and preparing for the handover of care to others.

The step by step methodology to achieve these goals is:

1. Using the "Saving the World, Saving Yourself" essay and *Working with Voices*, the mentor generates a discussion with the resident of unusual events that she or he has experienced prior to and possibly during the stay at the facility.

2. Through this discussion times of misperception of events are identified and the events are normalized as examples of confusion that are causing the person to not be able to get what he or she want out of life.

3. Using the cases of misperception, the mentor explains to the person the idea that people like them appear to be "vision quest prone" (or other terms that are part of the agreed-on vocabulary used to describe the experiences) and that as a result there have been and may continue to be times where she or he misperceive events and become confused.

4. The mentor points out the need for the person to reality check events and to review events with a person who will act as a sounding board to help avoid misperception. The mentor offers to be a sounding board for the person, promising to be as

confidential and trustworthy as possible, and encourages reality checking as a general habit.

5. The resident and the mentor begin a review of unusual events in the person's past (and possibly present) to identify triggers for events, underlying traumas that may be exacerbating the events and the meaning of significant events in the context of the person's life content and issues of concern. Means to minimize the unusual events are also determined. The toolkit is used to guide this process.

6. As the resident improves and accepts the idea of having a trusted other as a sounding board, the mentor has the resident identify people that they consider trustworthy who will be present in the resident's life after leaving the facility.

7. An agreement is made with at least one of these individuals to be a sounding board for the person after they leave the facility, allowing the discussion of past unusual events to continue and any new events to be identified.

8. A packet is prepared and given to the person acting as the new sounding board to pass on the key discoveries during this process and to allow a continuity of care for the resident.

At the same time, the staff should have two clear priorities for the family of the resident. First, the family should be ready to implement a plan to create an environment sensitive to the issues and triggers of returning resident, accept the resident pursuing her/his spiritual quest in mundane ways during recovery and either have one or more members act as trusted other for reality checking and being a sounding board or help resident maintain contact with trusted other(s) outside the family. Second, the mentor, the family members and the person in treatment should review the packet together at a meeting to begin to implement the new plan when the person is ready to leave the medium-term facility. This includes a plan to work with the individual(s) acting to check reality and be sounding boards for the person if outside the family.

APPENDIX C
POST-PSYCHOTIC SURVEYS

OVERVIEW

In 2011, I undertook a survey of people who self-identified as having experienced psychosis. The respondents were drawn from people in my own area and people I had met at conferences. I undertook the survey to seek to see if the salient characteristics of my own experiences were common to others who had also experienced the condition. By the late fall of 2011, I had received ten responses. Each respondent was given $20 for participating in the survey.

Though the survey was constructed for essay responses, most of the questions could be identified as being answered as "Yes" or "No." Following the guidance in methodology kindly given to me by Dr. Yegan Pillay of Ohio University, volunteers were recruited from local professionals working with, friends and family members of people with mental health challenges. These volunteers, without knowledge of the respondents, evaluated the survey answers on a question-by-question basis, determining if they believed the questions were being answered "Yes" or "No" and providing citation in the essay for their determination.

Each essay had three evaluators assigned to it. Evaluators read the essays separately and, after the essays had been read, evaluators met together to compare answers. Though discussion followed a structure, evaluators were encouraged to make additional comments, which included unsolicited statements about whether or not the person filling out the essay appeared to be still in psychosis. Of the ten essays, evaluators indicated the belief that four people were still in psychosis and that one person was actually describing a panic attack that was being shaded to fit the purpose of the survey. There was consensus among the evaluators and myself that the essay describing a panic attack should be thrown out, leaving nine essays.

In terms of evaluation of actual questions, two thirds of all evaluations resulted in all three evaluators agreeing prior to any discussion on a "Yes" or "No" answer. Another 13.5% of questions reached consensus through discussion, leaving just under 20% of the responses determined by a 2 to 1 vote or left undetermined. Evaluators remarked that reliability between their judgments seemed high.

In 2012, prior to completing the evaluation process, *Schizophrenia: A Blueprint for Recovery*, was published. Appendix C in the book contained my own, informal, evaluation of the surveys that was very close to the evaluations reached by the volunteers, excepting on the belief that four respondents were still psychotic. This important point is discussed below.

THEORETICAL APPROACH

The theoretical approach to this study is that people who experience psychosis are "vision quest prone." Vision quests, in cultures where they are recognized, are hallucinatory trance states often brought on intentionally by physical stress and deprivation. Vision quests are believed in these cultures to be communication with "other worlds" and to contain information relevant to the person and his or her community. Vision quests as such require attention and action to incorporate the lessons of the experience into the personal and community life of the person. An example of an accurate vision quest was the shaman Sitting Bull's prophetic vision of the Lakota victory over Custer during the Lakota Sun Dance ceremony.

For those who are vision quest prone, they may enter these hallucinatory states without realizing it and the state may grow in intensity and complexity over time. While there may be accurate intuitions during this state, the misinterpretation of hallucinatory events and metaphors for actual, literal events creates a set of odd beliefs outsiders think of as delusions. The experience may also cause the person to become highly mystical in response to actual and supposed events.

In terms of treatment, this view has three components.

1. Stop the hallucinatory events, either through stress reduction or medication (or both)
2. Return to the delusional framework and events during psychosis and discern actual or meaningful events from nonsensical events

3. Incorporate the implications of the actual or meaningful events into one's daily life

The questions asked in the survey are seeking to determine if the psychotic state mimics the conditions of the vision quest state.

THE RESULTS OF THE EVALUATIONS

I made the decision to throw out G-3, a respondent who evaluators felt was describing a panic attack and was shading answers to conform to survey questions. I concurred with this perspective.

It is my contention that the headline questions for each of the first five questions were initially supported by the findings from the remaining nine respondents. The numbers are as follows.

	YES	NO
Question 1: Real basis for beliefs?	6	3
Question 2: Ideas from outside sources?	8	1
Question 3: Stress triggering events?	7	2
Question 4: Magical or Spiritual Quest?	7	2
Question 5: Words with special meaning (made up or given)?	7	2

Please note that in Question 5 on connotative meanings of words, I indicate "Yes" if a respondent answered affirmatively to either "making up" or "giving" special meaning to words.

There are substantial implications for treatment should these numbers prove to hold up in larger trials. For example, if the proportions for question 4 and 5 hold to the normal population of people in psychosis, it would imply that more than 70% of the population believes that they are on a spiritual or magical quest to improve the world. An equal portion are using and interpreting language with special connotative meanings, a finding with implications for the symptom of "frequent derailment of or nonsensical" speech.

As a technical comment on the evaluation process, there are two questions that are a subset of Q1 that I should comment on.

	YES	NO
Did the person report accurate intuition?	4	5
Did the person report insights?	7	1

In the question on accurate intuition, though less than half of the evaluators noted statements affirming accurate intuitions during psychosis, I believe that this finding is important in indicating the possibility that despite the confused state of psychosis, for many people experiencing it there may be moments of heightened awareness that support the overall delusional framework. This has substantial implications for both treatment and analysis of this data. In this case, people who believe they are on a spiritual quest and are using language in a highly connotative manner may have accurate intuitions that occurred during psychosis that they believe support the validity of the quest and connotative meanings.

Second, on reported insights, I believe that my instructions to the evaluators were unclear on this question. The question was intended to discuss real life insights during psychosis that were not related to the recognition of psychosis itself. In some cases, evaluators answered affirmative when the respondent indicating insights after psychosis or about being psychotic, creating (I believe) some false positives.

Also significant are evaluator remarks on continuing to be delusional.

	YES	NO
Perceived as still delusional	4	5

When this subset is broken down, substantial implications to the findings are made both in terms of support of the findings and ability of individuals to recover.

	PERCEIVED AS DELUSIONAL		NOT PERCEIVED AS DELUSIONAL	
	YES	NO	YES	NO
Question 1: Real basis for beliefs?	4	0	2	3
Question 2: Ideas from outside sources?	4	0	4	1
Question 3: Stress triggering events?	2	2	5	0
Question 4: Magical or Spiritual Quest?	4	0	3	2
Question 5: Words with special meaning?	3	1	4	1

In this analysis, there is substantially more support in the still delusional group for a real basis to their beliefs, to stress as not being a triggering agent, and to being on a spiritual quest. Given this, the survey would seem to be indicating that these findings might be clustered in groups who have not truly recovered from their disease. However, relying on data from work history provided to me and not shared with the evaluators, the following data pattern appears (note: the work status of one respondent was not known, leaving eight respondents).

	DISABLED		WORKING	
	YES	NO	YES	NO
Question 1 Real basis for beliefs?	2	2	4	0
Question 2 Ideas from outside sources?	4	0	4	0
Question 3 Stress triggering events?	3	1	3	1
Question 4 Magical or Spiritual Quest?	2	2	4	0
Question 5 Words with special meaning?	3	1	3	1
Perceived as still delusional	1	3	3	1

In this finding, the perception of still being delusional is clustered with working full time. Most of those perceived as delusional were met at conferences on mental illness, and are employed full time as "Peer Specialists" in mental health organizations. It is also noteworthy that in the time since the essays, three individuals who were identified as "still delusional" all received state or national attention for their work in helping others recover. Given this, it appears that the perception of that these people are still delusional is not accurate.

It is my contention that the results actually support the overall theoretical view of psychosis as an unrecognized vision quest. The rationale is as follows. Since the psychotic state contains accurate and meaningful information relevant to the person's life, incorporating these experiences into the person's world view is a healthy part of the recovery process. This includes a possibility of an increase in highly mystical thinking, as is found in some forms of Catholicism, Hinduism, Buddhism, and other common world religions. From the outside point of view, these viewpoints may appear delusional; however, they are actually a recognition arising from the accurate portions of the psychotic experience.

A case in point is one respondent who indicated that he had switched spiritual traditions to neo-paganism, which is a highly mystical belief system that includes focus on accurate intuitions and oracles, trance states, and thought manifestation. He also takes medication to prevent recurrence of hallucinations. Despite having adopted these viewpoints and associating with others who share them, the respondent works full time and has been married for a number of years. According to the theoretical viewpoint, this is a healthy transformation of beliefs arising from the accurate and meaningful experiences of their hallucinatory journey.

It is important to note that the perception of respondents still being delusional was not part of the original evaluation, but rather was the results of spontaneous comments on the part of evaluators. Future surveys like these would benefit from formally including this question to evaluators while shielding evaluators from information like work status which can measure functionality.

DETAILED RESULTS OF EVALUATION

SUMMARY OF RESULTS	YES	NO
Question 1 Real basis for beliefs?	6	3
Question 2 Ideas from outside sources?	8	1
Question 3 Stress triggering events?	7	2
Question 4 Magical or Spiritual Quest?	7	2
Question 5 Words with special meaning (made up or given)?	7	2

DETAILED RESULTS	*YES*	*NO*
Question 1		
Did this person indicate that real events supported their belief in the psychosis?	6	3
Did the person report accurate intuition?	4	5
Did the person report insights?	7	1
Did the person report symbolic or metaphorical beliefs?	5	3
Did the person report coincidental events?	5	4

DETAILED RESULTS	YES	NO
Question 2		
Did the person indicate that ideas came from outside sources?	8	1
Did the person report ideas from the media?	6	3
Did the person report ideas from books?	6	3
Did the person report ideas from the internet?	0	9
Question 3		
Did the person report stress as triggering hallucinations or delusions?	7	2
Question 4		
Did the person report being on a magical or spiritual quest?	7	2
Question 5		
Did the person report making up words or phrases with special meanings?	3	6
Did the person report giving words or phrases special meanings?	7	2
Did the person report these words/phrases having special power?	5	4

APPENDIX D
STIGMA AND BEING A SENSITIVE PERSON

I am a sensitive person, prone to strong vulnerable feelings such as love, hope, sorrow, regret, enjoyment of beauty and desires for a better human world. I treasure my growth as a person to be a nice person to be best of my limited ability, and find the typical view of manhood as filled with senseless aggression and empty bravado. As a sensitive person, I believe the most important thing I can do is be a good husband and step-father. The second most important thing I can do is to walk gently on this Earth, respecting others and seeking to do as little harm to all life, human and otherwise, as I can. And while these are my ideals, on a day to day basis I often fail to be kind, loving and appreciative of the many good people and aspects of my life that I am mysteriously fortunate to be gifted by.

In writing this, I am aware that I am someone who has repeatedly received miraculous help, sometimes from strangers, sometimes from blind luck and most of all by people—mainly women—who have gone out of their way to care for me when I was in dire need. As a recipient of these gifts—as well as many others—I have repeatedly been given not only a renewed life but a sense of joyous recognition of a spiritual life as a daily companion. Because of these things, I have a very fortunate life and have had many years of happiness that many people—in the mental health subculture or not—have not experienced. Without these things, it would be much harder for me to be sensitive, to be comfortable in my manhood and to be able to enjoy my quiet life with my family and small community.

In speaking about stigma, it is important for me to talk about what I like about myself, because stigma, especially self-stigma, is being victimized by feelings of not being worthy and likable. I like being sensitive, including at this time in my middle age as a man who often "gets weepy" when thinking of happy times with young children, the good people I know, my wife and family and a number of other things. I treasure my softness, my desire not to argue and my experience that the more that I have tried to do good works to help others the more I have received kindness and support from others.

It is this sensitivity that is so important to my view of myself as a schizophrenic, because I believe that I am a schizophrenic because I am a sensitive person who experienced trauma early in life. This combination resulted in psychosis. I am grateful for being a schizophrenic because it helped me regain my sensitivity and made all the good things in my life possible. In doing so, I recognize that in my life I have actually encountered more stigma as a sensitive man than as someone who is public about being schizophrenic. In my case, I also see schizophrenia as a sort of proto-personality marked by deep feelings, sensitivity, abstraction and idealism, that when mixed with various traumas results in what is called psychosis. From this vantage point, both sensitivity and schizophrenia are gifts that have made my life better. The damage that succumbing to self-stigma would do is to cause me to reject my liking being a sensitive person and a schizophrenic.

When I first accepted that I was a schizophrenic, I talked about being proud of being schizophrenic. This must sound odd to people who think, consciously or unconsciously, that it is bad to be what I am, and I chose to say "proud" because I wanted to make it clear that being a schizophrenic is not something I have any shame in being. As I have matured, I have become increasingly aware that virtually all of my qualities have been gifts given me by people and things outside myself. From my vantage point, to take pride in anything I am or have is nonsensical because it is not something I truly am, it is something I have been gifted to receive. Pride also is a consciousness that separates me from others, setting myself apart from and above others. This is a highly deceptive and dangerous consciousness because it makes me, in the end, isolated from the lives around me. It creates an "I-and-other" view of the world, rather than a "we" view of the world, estranging me from the spirit that I witness in daily life.

My feelings about being a schizophrenic have not changed, but my feelings about pride have. So I now say, "I like being a schizophrenic" or more gently, "I am glad I have schizophrenia" because for me this is synonymous with being a sensitive person. This doesn't mean that schizophrenia or sensitivity are entirely positive things, because in my experience, everything and everyone are mixtures of positive and negative qualities. But for me, I am as much grateful for my journey through psychosis as a rugged cowboy is fond of his best horse. I would not be who I am, or sharing my life with those I now dearly love, were it not for the bizarre, life threatening events that occurred to me some 30 years ago. Schizophrenia is the horse that took me from being a person whose sensitivity was buried under layers of trauma across a treacherous stream of self-awakening into a new, happier and much more authentic life.

In recognizing that there are negative qualities in all things, including what we call psychosis and schizophrenia (or "madness" if you prefer), it is important to attempt to turn weaknesses into strengths. To do this, we must face our weaknesses, our shadow elements, and transform them. To discuss this and its implications in the mental health arena, I want to include a substantial section from a report I wrote summarizing my experiences at several conferences in 2011.

I. Most major behavioral advances are innovations by family members and peers

Newly established and cutting edge advances in behavioral means to work with mental illnesses (Dialectical Behavioral Therapy; Wellness Recovery Action Plan; Listen-Empathize-Agree-Partner; CommonGround Software and Personal Medicine) are the achievements of mentally ill people and family members. Of the behavioral therapies I have been exposed to, only Cognitive Behavioral Therapy has been advanced by academics and clinicians not directly affected by mental illness. This reveals that for the past several decades stakeholders (peers and family members) have been contributing substantially to the recovery model while academicians and clinicians have lagged behind.

II. Problems in communication between clinicians, family members, and peers

Despite the achievement of peers and family members, there is a marked lack of communication between different groups within the subculture. Very few clinicians and academicians attend conferences and presentations by family members and mentally ill people. Very few family members attend peer conferences. I argue that this lack of interest in exchanges of information is the greatest obstacle to rapid advances in the recovery movement.

III. Internal feuding between peers and family members hampers delivery of diversity of services

Despite common goals of fostering recovery, at the national level peers and family members are feuding about differing treatment modalities, making cooperation difficult. This debate is centered primarily on medication verses non-medication as a treatment approach. Underlying this debate is a game of hot-potato with stigma. Family members refuse to acknowledge any contribution to stresses and failures of recovery of mentally ill family members, framing the discussion in terms of chemical imbalances; peers often refuse to acknowledge personal failings and discussion of diagnosis and surrounding behaviors, making the process of turning weaknesses into strengths more difficult. Everyone has faults and flaws; peers and family members often approach the treatment arena with a denial of this basic fact. By refusing to acknowledge shortcomings on all sides, many complementary treatment approaches are unfairly polarized around debates on medication that contain hidden agendas aimed at not acknowledging ways that we all can negatively impact recovery.

IV. Need for peers/family members to work closely together

To overcome the problems of communication blocks and failure to provide a menu of diverse treatment modalities as part of recovery options, it is essential that organizations of peers and family members work closely together. A primary goal of this should be to educate academicians and clinicians on the many new treatment approaches being created by mentally ill people and their family members and engage these professionals in studying and popularizing the achievements of peers and family members.

V. Family member and peer inability to simultaneously face personal failings and maintain self-love creates false self-esteem that interferes with recovery

At the core of conflict between family member and peer feuds is a false form of self-esteem, common in our culture, that to be worthy at all one needs to be without flaw. Accordingly, people strive to put forward the image, especially to ourselves, that we are without failing and therefore worthy of respect. This is in complete denial of my own personal experience that almost everyone I have known personally had times of personal failures; many fail to admit their failings, complicating the harm they do/have done. Progress on resolving the stigma hot-potato debate requires a true model of self-esteem which maintains that people are lovable and have many redeeming qualities despite having major failings that require personal work to grow psychologically and spiritually—i.e., improving our relationships with each other.

If we are to be concerned about stigma, the first step is to reject self-stigma that maintains that because we are peers/consumers/survivors/schizophrenics/etc. that somehow we are to believe we are more grievously flawed than others. Everyone I know, whether they have schizophrenia like I do or not, have had times of tremendous personal failing. Many people I know refuse to face their character flaws, causing the problems to fester and rot away at their lives. If we are to not be destroyed by the negative aspects of our condition, we need to face them squarely while still believing we are worthy of love by others and ourselves. For that reason I prefer to call myself a schizophrenic. This confronts stigma and self-stigma in the face. If someone does not like me because I am what I am, it is his or her problem to deal with, not mine.

Changing stigma in others is much more complex than changing it in ourselves, but we must change it in ourselves first. We must give up the false self-esteem in which we refuse to admit we have faults and instead nurture a real sense within us that it is okay to be flawed because we still have good qualities. Once we do this, we can turn our mind to building on our good qualities while reducing our negative ones. This helps our spiritual journey by making us better people, improving our relationships with others and strengthening the web of life around us.

In our spiritual journey it is essential to take responsibility for our adult lives, including our choices to enter and stay in situations. Whether abuse, addiction, illness, harming others or other problems, we must always ask ourselves, "Why did I enter into and stay in this situation?" We need to ask ourselves why we entered into situations, both good and bad, and who influenced us to make these choices. Even when the answer is that we were acting in response to trauma or under duress, such questions allow us to recognize what we need to do to avoid bad situations and enter into good ones. This gives us a chance to empower ourselves and improve our lives.

In terms of self-stigma within peers, probably my greatest concern is the failure to see psychosis as being both a spiritually-uplifting experience and a condition that threatens the life and well-being ourselves as well as others. It is important to avoid thinking of psychosis as "bad" and follow the logic that "bad creates bad" and "good creates good." If we do, we arrive at the belief that trauma creates psychosis and both trauma and psychosis are bad things that result from one another. If psychosis is only a product of the bad experience of trauma then its value as an unrecognized vision quest is lost. If it is only a good experience, then we never have to take responsibility for our negative acts during psychosis.

By seeing the good and bad in all things, including in psychosis and in ourselves, we can overcome self-stigma and see how our experiences can both benefit and cause problems for people. We liberate ourselves from false self-esteem that dictates that we hide our flaws from ourselves. We can love ourselves enough to recognize both our virtues and our imperfections, including our severe character flaws. This allows us to build on our strengths while lessening our negative qualities and their impact on others. Such a mentally healthy approach holds the potential for us to become better people both within ourselves and in how we treat others. If we can do this we will overcome both our self-stigma and the stigma that is given to us by outsiders.

Appendix E
Websites of Interest

THE MEDICATION DEBATE

Robert Whitaker

https://www.madinamerica.com/

Paris Williams

http://www.rethinkingmadness.com/

Ron Coleman

http://www.roncolemanvoices.co.uk/

http://www.workingtorecovery.co.uk/

E. Fuller Torrey

http://www.treatmentadvocacycenter.org/

THE COMBINED TOOLKIT

Paris Williams

http://www.rethinkingmadness.com/

Ron Coleman

http://www.roncolemanvoices.co.uk/

http://www.workingtorecovery.co.uk/

Hearing Voices Network – USA

http://www.hearingvoicesusa.org/

LEAP

http://www.leapinstitute.org/

WRAP

http://www.mentalhealthrecovery.com/wrap/

Open Dialogue

http://willhall.net/opendialogue/

http://www.dialogicpractice.net/

CBT

http://www.nacbt.org/

Common Ground and Personal Medicine

https://www.patdeegan.com/

EMDR

http://www.emdr.com/

Re-Evaluation Counseling

https://www.rc.org/

eCPR

http://www.emotional-cpr.org/

SUPPORT ORGANIZATIONS

National Alliance on Mental Illness

http://www.nami.org/

Depression Bipolar Support Alliance

http://www.dbsalliance.org/

Mother Bear

http://motherbearcan.com/

Recovering Our Families courses

http://family.practicerecovery.com/

Schizophrenics Anonymous

http://www.sardaa.org/

National Empowerment Center

http://www.power2u.org/

ADDITIONAL WEBSITES

CooperRiis Healing Community

http://www.cooperriis.org/

Prescription for Nutritional Healing

http://prescriptionfornutritionalhealing.net/

Alcoholics Anonymous

http://www.aa.org/

Al-Anon and Alateen

http://www.al-anon.alateen.org/

About Milt Greek

Milt Greek is a husband and stepfather of adult children and has worked as a computer programmer since the fall of 1989. When he was in college as a psychology major and sociology graduate student, Milt developed psychosis, resulting in repeated hospitalizations and severe damage to his academic work. After returning to sanity through the help of friends, family, professionals and medication, Milt finished his degrees but retrained to find work.

Milt has had a very fortunate and full life, with a happy marriage and a quiet life in a small college town. Beginning in the mid-1990s, Milt volunteered with a few people in acute psychosis as well as founding a peer early recovery group for people with schizophrenia. In the late 1990s, Milt began to speak at conferences on schizophrenia and recovery, as well as initiating research into psychosis through subject-participant groups and a small survey of people in post-psychosis. Beginning in 2007, Milt began workshops training professionals in understanding and working with people in psychosis and post-psychosis. In 2009, Milt recorded DVDs and created a website to host them. His first book, *Schizophrenia: A Blueprint for Recovery* was published in 2011, with a revised edition published in 2012.

In 2014, after nearly 20 years of volunteering and working in the area of psychosis and recovery while maintaining a full-time job and pursuing several other outside projects,

Milt began a lengthy sabbatical from mental health work to spend more time with his wife and family and pursue other projects. Though the website hosting his material was discontinued, the material on the website is contained in the two books Milt has written on this topic.

Though the sabbatical is planned for an indefinite length of time, Milt wishes the best to all people affected by the hardships of life: "Regardless of the nature of our challenges, we are all united in our struggle to celebrate life in the face of the deaths of those we love, including ourselves. May we all experience the joy of being loved and being able to love in this hard and wonderful world."

Made in the USA
Lexington, KY
22 September 2015